Sole Guidance

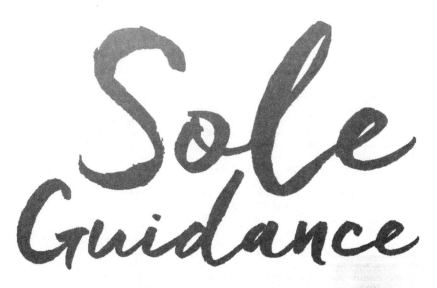

Sole Guidance

ANCIENT SECRETS *of* CHINESE REFLEXOLOGY *to* HEAL *the* BODY, MIND, HEART, *and* SPIRIT

Holly Tse

HAY HOUSE, INC.
Carlsbad, California • New York City
London • Sydney • Johannesburg
Vancouver • New Delhi

Published and distributed in the United States by: Hay House, Inc.: www.hayhouse .com • **Published and distributed in Australia by:** Hay House Australia Pty. Ltd.: www.hayhouse.com.au • **Published and distributed in the United Kingdom by:** Hay House UK, Ltd.: www.hayhouse.co.uk • **Published and distributed in the Republic of South Africa by:** Hay House SA (Pty), Ltd.: www.hayhouse.co.za • **Distributed in Canada by:** Raincoast Books: www.raincoast.com • **Published in India by:** Hay House Publishers India: www.hayhouse.co.in

Cover design: Michelle Polizzi • *Interior design:* Pamela Homan
Illustrations by © Holly Tse, www.ChineseFootReflexology.com

Library of Congress Cataloging-in-Publication Data

Names: Tse, Holly, date, author.
Title: Sole guidance : ancient secrets of Chinese reflexology to heal the
  body, mind, heart, and spirit / Holly Tse.
Description: 1st edition. | Carlsbad, California : Hay House, Inc., 2016.
Identifiers: LCCN 2016014318 | ISBN 9781401949273 (paperback)
Subjects: LCSH: Reflexotherapy. | Foot--Massage. | BISAC: HEALTH & FITNESS /
  Alternative Therapies. | HEALTH & FITNESS / Massage & Reflexotherapy. |
  BODY, MIND & SPIRIT / Healing / Energy (Chi Kung, Reiki, Polarity).
Classification: LCC RM723.R43 T74 2016 | DDC 615.8/224--dc23 LC record avail-
able at https://lccn.loc.gov/2016014318

ISBN: 978-1-4019-4927-3
10 9 8 7 6 5 4 3 2 1
1st edition, July 2016

Printed in the United States of America

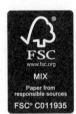

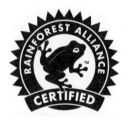

CONTENTS

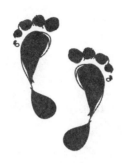

Your Journey Begins

An Important Note

Within this book, I share information about how to locate and massage Chinese reflexology points. Please note that if you are pregnant, it is recommended that you do not practice reflexology as there are acupuncture points in the feet and near the ankles that are used to induce labor. In addition, if you have an acute heart condition, it is best to avoid practicing reflexology.

Please note that the recommendations may or may not be appropriate for you. Please check with your physician, health-care professional, or therapist prior to starting any new health regimen.

CHAPTER 1

Three Catalysts for Health and Vitality

As a second generation Chinese Canadian, I was raised to do well in school and get a good job. I dutifully followed this program as best I could, even though I knew in my heart that I was meant to follow a different path.

When I was six years old, my teacher asked the class what we wanted to be when we grew up. The other kids said things like fireman, nurse, and astronaut. I wrote down that I wanted to be a *loyer*. I remember being very confused when Mrs. Smith gently corrected me and spelled the word out loud: "L-A-W-Y-E-R." How could that be the right spelling for my chosen career?

When I was 13, it dawned on me that I had no idea what a lawyer was and that I really didn't want to be one. I was drawn to art and design, but never thought I could do what I loved for a living. My mom would tell me, "Your cousin is good at art, but it's a *hobby*. That's why he is studying computers."

I thought a good compromise would be to get a business degree and work in marketing. My first job out of university lasted for six months before the boredom forced me to quit. I stayed at my second job for two and a half years, but I had an exit plan in place even before my first day of work. I always felt like I had to put in my time before I could do what I wanted to.

It became a pattern that I would start a new job and like it until I had mastered the tasks. After that, I would get bored and stick it out until I couldn't take it any longer. In between jobs, I gave myself permission to follow my heart and pursue interests I loved, but because my mind was so dominant, that didn't last very long. I always returned to the corporate world. I kept trying to change my circumstances within the confines of having a "good" job.

This went on for over 15 years. I would sit at my office desk, yet every cell in my body would be screaming at me to get up and walk out the door. I forced myself to stay because my mind was calling all the shots. I had a good job and was making good money in the "glamorous" field of web design. I worked on high-profile projects for some of the biggest consumer brands in the world.

By society's standards, I was highly successful. People *aspired* to have my career, so what right did I have to say it wasn't good enough for me? How could I walk away from a "perfect" career because I was unhappy and my life felt meaningless?

Over time, doing something I despised every day took a toll on my health and well-being. My body protested by breaking down, and my thoughts turned negative, filled with resentment, anger, and hopelessness. Outwardly, I seemed reasonably calm, but inside I was seething. I blamed "incompetent" co-workers for making my job more difficult. I blamed managers for failing to support me. I blamed my job for my unhappiness. Looking back, though, there was no reason to blame anyone—not even myself. All I had to do was simply walk away.

When you ignore your soul's calling, the Universe steps in to help you along. At first, it lights a path for you to follow. The path may not be entirely clear at the beginning, but as long as you step forward, you continue to be guided. However, when you dismiss the signs, the Universe gets your attention in ways that you can't ignore.

For me, my work environment would always deteriorate. All sorts of drama and trauma would bubble up until I felt like I was forced to quit. However, I kept going back for more.

There was only one thing that made me pay attention, and that was when my body broke down and my health suffered. As a result, over the course of ten years, I experienced three major health crises. With each crisis, I discovered a catalyst to heal my body, and each catalyst was more powerful than the previous.

The third catalyst was so powerful that it not only restored my health, it enabled me to thrive. I felt stronger, healthier, happier, and more alive than I had in years. And there was an extra bonus that came with the third catalyst—I found my life purpose.

The First Catalyst

In my mid-20s, I was in a car accident that left me with chronic pain in my neck and shoulders. The car was struck from the side by another vehicle. Unfortunately, I was sitting on the side that took the brunt of the impact. I felt like my body was broken and I would be doomed to suffer for the rest of my life. Before the accident, Dan, my boyfriend at the time, and I had planned to do a cross-Canada bicycle trip. After the accident, I rarely rode my bike as it was too much of a strain on my upper body, and I was also afraid of injuring myself further.

One day, Dan turned to me and asked if we were still going to ride our bikes across Canada. He knew we wouldn't be doing it right away, but wondered if it might be something we would do in the future. The word *no* was on the tip of my tongue when I heard a voice inside me say, *If you say no, this car accident will define you for the rest of your life.*

So instead, I said, "Yes, let's try it. If I have any problems with my neck, we can always catch a bus home." In that moment,

I discovered the first catalyst for healing my body—*shifting the mind.*

That one decision completely altered the course of my life. If I had said *no,* I would have chosen a lifetime of limitations. When I said *yes,* the accident no longer held power over me.

I realized that I had blindly accepted other people's beliefs about chronic pain. My body didn't need to ache when it rained. I didn't have to suffer for life because of old scar tissue. I had the power to choose differently for myself.

As a result, I became open to the possibility that I could live a life free from pain. When I accepted others' beliefs without question, I felt like I was "ruined" for the rest of my life. As a result, I didn't have the motivation or inspiration to look beyond my comfort zone for solutions. After all, why would you look for a cure when you believe there is none? However, once I let go of the limitations, I was open to seeking new knowledge, and I started reaching out to people outside of my network for help—and that's what led me to alternative healing. My outlook brightened, my attitude improved, and I found the people who could help me heal my body.

About a year and a half after the accident, Dan and I went on our cross-Canada bike trip. We started in Vancouver and rode over 2,000 miles across mountains and prairies back to Dan's hometown in northern Ontario. Throughout the entire journey, I did not experience a single problem with my neck or shoulders.

Our final destination was his parents' home, where we were greeted with a delicious blueberry pie freshly baked by his mom. It was the *best* blueberry pie ever. While Dan and I ended up parting ways a few years after the bicycle trip, we remained good friends and still reminisce fondly about the trip.

The Second Catalyst

After the bicycle trip, I felt so free that I gave myself the freedom to do things that I enjoyed. I taught myself how to build websites and started a self-published online magazine that gained quite a following, and even got me featured in a university textbook. I decided to change careers and work in the Internet industry. However, I was ignoring the voice inside me that called me toward the field of healing.

Working in high tech was extremely stressful. The timelines were tight, the clients demanding, and employees were expected to devote their lives to their jobs. My health was fine for several years, but the chronic stress gradually eroded my resilience. After working at an exceptionally demanding company that exponentially amped my stress levels, I experienced what I refer to as my *year of illness*. I was afflicted by one weird ailment or disease after another. The doctors told me I was perfectly healthy, but I knew there was something wrong.

When I reached the lowest point in my health, my husband, Zunaid, suggested I go see his Chinese reflexologist. Even though I embraced alternative healing, I was entirely skeptical. I asked him, "Isn't that where they rub your feet? How is that going to help me?"

The first time I received a Chinese reflexology treatment, I was in tears. I quickly realized this wasn't the low cost "happy lucky foot massage" that you see in tiny shops dotting Chinatown. This was *real* Chinese reflexology.

All of the reflexology points on my feet were extremely sensitive, which indicated that I had major energy disharmonies in all of my organs. After the first session, I didn't want to go back. However, Zunaid and I had made a deal where I would see his reflexologist for a month if he would go see my naturopath.

As I received regular reflexology sessions over the course of a couple of months, my health stabilized. And then when I started studying Chinese reflexology and practicing on myself, my health improved even further.

I learned that the traditional Chinese method of reflexology differed significantly from the Western style. Aside from being way more intense, Chinese reflexology was based on the principles of Traditional Chinese Medicine (TCM)—an ancient healing system that encompasses acupuncture, energy healing, Chinese herbs, and massage.

Chinese reflexology is a niche within Chinese Medicine. If you consider acupuncture to be a branch of TCM, then Chinese reflexology would be a twig. However, it works a lot like acupuncture, only without the needles. By massaging pressure points on your feet, you balance the energy meridians, also referred to as channels, in your body. These channels are a circulatory system for *qi* (pronounced "chee"), your life force energy. When there are problems in your body, the flow of qi is disrupted. By harmonizing your qi, you help your body return to a state of balance, too.

It certainly worked for me. Less than a year and a half after hitting rock bottom, I felt so good that I was training for my first triathlon. I had discovered the second catalyst for healing my body—*healing with energy.*

Chinese reflexology gave me the power to know what was going at the energy level, so that I could turn things around before they manifested at the physical level. When work became even more stressful than usual, I could feel the effects on my body as I massaged the reflexology points on my feet. One by one, I observed my organs going off-line energetically. And that's what finally prompted me to quit my job and seriously consider doing what I loved.

Of course, I hadn't counted on how stubborn my mind was . . .

The Third Catalyst

After I left my job, I started writing a book on DIY cat toys (*Make Your Own Cat Toys: Saving the Planet One Cat Toy at a Time*), and I also began seeing reflexology clients. Things were going really well, but my mind couldn't resist the lure of a full-time job. I was so conditioned by society and my Asian upbringing that I felt compelled to work in the corporate world. I was tempted by a high-tech position in Silicon Valley and convinced myself that relocating to sunny California with its laid-back attitude would be different from my previous pattern.

Once again, work started off great. The project was interesting and my co-workers were awesome. People actually left their desks to eat lunch. I could even wear flip flops to work!

The honeymoon lasted for a few months, but storm clouds were brewing. Over the course of two years, my division was reorganized four times within the company, I had five different managers, and our business direction went from building for long-term growth to putting out fires for short-term gains. The work environment deteriorated so drastically that in the time that I was there, I went from being the newbie in my department to the employee with the longest tenure.

In my previous jobs, I had found it challenging to do the same thing every day for years. However, the projects and clients had always been changing, and I'd been given a great deal of autonomy and responsibility. Now that I was working for a large corporation, everything felt so bureaucratic. The work was menial and every decision I made had to be reviewed by over 20 people. I was micromanaged, underappreciated, and completely demotivated.

When I moved to California, I was hopeful that I could work full-time in high tech and continue to pursue my passion for healing part-time. However, as my workweek ballooned to 50-plus hours and the job sucked the life out of me, I no longer had the energy to practice Chinese reflexology on friends and family. I even stopped massaging my own feet.

At the office, I would sit in front of my computer screen and literally think, *I can't stand staring at this screen all day. I can't stand what I'm looking at.*

My body heard my thoughts and responded. I began having problems with my vision where I would suddenly be unable to see. It was as if a hundred camera flashes went off before my eyes. I couldn't read, I couldn't focus, and I certainly couldn't use the computer. The disorientation lasted for about 30 minutes, and afterward I was completely exhausted.

I was diagnosed with ocular migraines. My optometrist told me there was no cure and the cause was unknown. The best thing I could do was to avoid the triggers—fluorescent lighting, computer screens, and bright sunlight—all the things that were a major part of my life.

The optometrist also told me that I had signs of early-stage macular degeneration. This eye disease causes sufferers to lose the central portion of their vision. According to Western medicine, there is no cure.

While most people develop this disease in their senior years, I was in my mid-30s when the eye doctor gave me the diagnosis. In my heart, I knew it was because my body was responding to my thoughts: *I can't stand what I'm looking at.*

Perhaps that's why I didn't immediately panic about the prospect of losing my eyesight. Truth be told, I was also preoccupied by the immediate issue of the ocular migraines. But there was also that spark in my heart that knew if my thoughts had created this disease, then I could change my thoughts to heal my body.

The upside of this experience was that it finally made me leave my career for good. I thought, *these are my eyes. I can't keep doing what I'm doing. I can't lose my vision.*

It was time to do what I wanted to do.

After years of being ruled by my mind, I made the decision to follow my heart, and it led me back to the path of healing. My life transformed almost overnight. Things that used to be a struggle became effortless. I used to work so hard trying to figure out what my life purpose was and to make it work as a career. However, when I listened to my heart, I simply *knew* what I needed to do in order to move forward—one step at a time. As I began seeing with the clarity of my heart, my energy levels soared and I completely healed my vision. And that was when I realized the third catalyst for health and vitality—*following your heart and soul.*

My Dragon Spirit

After I started listening to my heart and soul, I discovered that I could channel guidance from the Universe to help me follow my life purpose. I did this by sitting quietly in the dark and asking questions out loud. Then I would allow whatever words came to mind to flow through me. I even went so far as to speak them out loud.

During one of my channeling sessions, I was directed to call this guidance *Dragon Spirit*. Everyone has a Dragon Spirit within. It is not an entity or spirit outside of yourself. Instead, it is the voice inside you that craves adventure, exploration, excitement, and expression—and very conveniently, it has the most expansive answers to all of your questions.

Quite serendipitously, I discovered I could channel guidance to help other people, too. One day, I was speaking with a new friend on the phone, and we got on the topic of reincarnation and past lives. I shared with her that I had the experience of recalling a few past lives. She, on the other hand, had always wanted to remember a past life, but had been unable to do so, despite working with a couple of professionals to assist her.

It was then that my Dragon Spirit whispered to me, *Tell her you'll help her.* I was stunned. I had no clue on how to guide someone to revisit a past life, but my Dragon Spirit was insistent: *Tell her you'll help her now!*

So I asked my friend if she wanted to explore this with me, and she was excited to try. At first, I was grasping for what to say, but as I calmed down, the words just flowed through me. Within 15 minutes, my friend was in a deep state of relaxation and recounting details from a past life. I remember her giggling out loud as she exclaimed, "We have dogs!"

After that first spontaneous session for a friend, I continued channeling Dragon Spirit for others. I became much more comfortable with speaking the words that flowed through me, and I discovered that I could help people uncover their life purpose in just a few sessions, even if it had been eluding them for years. Dragon Spirit enables me to connect with people's energy. It lets me know what to say so that my clients can set aside their strong and powerful minds in order to hear their own Dragon Spirit. When clients are connected with their higher guidance, they have entered the Dragon Spirit space.

At first, I kept Dragon Spirit separate from my Chinese reflexology practice. However, when I noticed people gaining insights into long-standing health issues during their Dragon Spirit sessions, I became curious. I wondered what would happen if I combined it with reflexology.

The results were amazing. Clients healed faster when we delved into the emotional roots of their challenges rather than working with just the reflexology alone. People came to see me for health concerns, but also experienced deep emotional clearing and healing.

Looking back on my life, I once wondered why I had to experience so many health crises during my adulthood. My Dragon Spirit responded, *You have to experience them in order to teach them.*

I had found my soul's calling.

If I could go back in time and do things over, I'm not sure if I would change a thing, as I wouldn't have discovered the three catalysts for healing. These catalysts changed my life, and together they unlock the secrets to health, vitality, and leading a joyful life. I wake up full of excitement to face the day, and I live a life filled with immense joy and abundance.

It feels awesome to feel awesome, which is why I'm so passionate about sharing what I've learned with you. This book is the first of its kind to teach *authentic* Chinese reflexology in a way that is accessible for *everyone* to use in their day-to-day lives. What you're about to learn is the *real deal* for improving your health and wellness. And you can now discover the incredible secrets of this ancient, powerful healing practice from the comfort of your own home.

I'm so excited because it is my wish for you to live your passion and experience amazing health and vitality, too. If you know that your health could be better or that your life could be happier, then I invite you to join me on a journey of healing, exploration, and possibility. Perhaps this book is the Universe lighting a path for *you* to follow.

As Lao-tzu, the renowned Chinese philosopher, wrote in the *Tao Te Ching*, "A journey of a thousand miles begins with a single step."

Let your journey begin.

CHAPTER 2

You Are Here

Did you know that your feet are a source of wisdom? They reveal where you hold stress and how you approach life, and they can even tell you where emotional pain is hidden deep inside your body. Your feet never lie. They always tell the truth about your current state of health and well-being.

Chinese reflexology points on your feet correspond to different areas of your body. By checking the sensitivity of the reflexology points on your feet, you can gain insight into what is going on in your body.

Your feet can also give you insights on how to create harmony in your life, as well as clues for following your soul purpose. By listening to your feet, you can feel more connected with your body so that you can integrate your body, mind, heart, and spirit.

But before you begin your journey, it's important to get a snapshot of where you are right now. When you know where you're starting from, it can help you reach your destination faster.

It's like when you're at the mall looking at the directory and you're trying to figure out how to get to the shoe store. The map is overwhelming with all of those little boxes, squinty numbers, and an endless list of stores in categories that are too numerous to decipher.

However, once you see that little red dot with the words "You Are Here," you feel a sense of relief. Suddenly getting where you need to go becomes much easier. The same is true for healing your body and following your passion.

We are inundated with so much information that it's hard to know what is right. And don't even get me started about the Internet! It's the virtual candy store for the mind when it comes to researching what ails you.

Fortunately, there's a simple way to cut through the clutter. There are *three Chinese reflexology points* that can tell you what's going on in your body right now and what you can do to improve your health and vitality. By testing these points on your feet, you bypass your mind and get the truth straight from the best source of insider information—your body.

When you listen to your body, you begin realizing your own power to heal and transform your life. It is not the doctor, diet, or medication that heals—sure, they can help you along, but it really is your body that does the healing. That's why it's so important to pay attention to what your body has to say.

There's a Chinese proverb that says, *"The superior doctor prevents sickness. The mediocre doctor attends to impending sickness. The inferior doctor treats actual sickness."*

What this means is that a great doctor will help you stay healthy, whereas someone less skilled will allow things to progress until physical symptoms appear and then they will treat the condition at the early stage. On the other hand, an unskilled doctor will let things get so bad that you actually get sick, and then they will try to fix things.

This proverb makes it easy to blame the doctor when you get sick. However, it's very disempowering to do this. The old Chinese proverb needs to be tweaked for modern times. Here's my take on it:

"The superior patient prevents sickness. The mediocre patient attends to impending sickness. The inferior patient treats actual sickness. The really inferior patient sticks their head in the sand until things are so bad, it's almost (but not quite) impossible to return to wellness."

Unfortunately, it's pretty common in our modern society to ignore the early warning signs in our bodies. The mediocre patient will let things progress until they notice early-stage symptoms and then they will finally do something about it. The inferior patient lets things deteriorate to the point where they get completely sidelined before they address the problem.

And then, we have the really inferior patient who ignores the problem until they come down with something that is "incurable" or becomes chronic. At this point, the condition is much harder to treat, and it takes a much longer time to return to health.

So, my question for you is, who do you want to be? Regardless of what is going on in your body right now, you can be the superior patient—only you shouldn't see yourself as only a patient. When you do, you're giving away responsibility for your health. To take command of your health, you need to be your own "superior doctor," healing at the energy level to prevent physical symptoms *before* they happen.

If you can catch and reverse problems at the energy level, you can prevent them from manifesting in the physical body. For physical issues, you can also use healing at the energy level to support and superboost your body's natural healing process for a quicker return to wellness.

Massaging a reflexology point sends healing qi to the affected area, and this helps to improve the flow of blood to the area. In this way, qi supports the body in clearing toxins and getting what it needs to heal—whether it's oxygen, nutrients, or antibodies.

To figure out where your body needs healing energy the most, let's do a quick test of a few key Chinese reflexology points. Testing these points can uncover qi disharmonies in your body and also give you instant feedback on your overall health and well-being.

PLEASE NOTE IF YOU ARE PREGNANT

There are acupuncture points in and around your feet that are used to induce labor. Thus, it is best to avoid practicing reflexology on yourself if you are pregnant.

---

1. Chinese Reflexology Point for the Kidneys

Use It to Check: Your overall levels of life force qi.

Why It Matters: In Traditional Chinese Medicine, the Kidneys are considered the *root of life*. They store *Kidney jing*—your reserves of life force energy. The Kidneys are like batteries storing the energy available to you for your lifetime. When your Kidney jing is depleted, it's like draining the battery on your cell phone. Eventually, your phone dies, and the same thing happens to your body when you've used up all of your jing.

In Traditional Chinese Medicine, deficiency in the Kidneys is associated with numerous health issues:

- Exhaustion and chronic fatigue
- Fertility issues, low sex drive
- Premature aging: gray hair, weak knees, lower backache, hearing loss, and memory loss
- Edema
- Frequent urination
- Asthma and allergies

How to Test Your Kidney Reflexology Point

IMPORTANT

The Chinese reflexology point for the Kidney is quite close to the acupuncture point *Kidney 1*. This point is sometimes used to induce labor in a pregnant woman who is past her due date. Therefore, without proper training and extensive hands-on experience in locating these points, do not massage this point or practice reflexology on yourself if you are pregnant.

The Kidney point is an oval located on the sole of your foot. You have a Kidney point on each foot, but for this exercise, you'll use your left foot. We'll go over a simple method to get a general location for your Kidney point, and then we will take a more detailed approach later in this book.

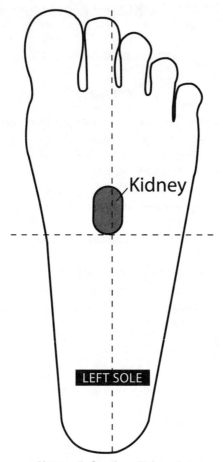

Chinese Reflexology Kidney Point

To locate the Kidney point, sit comfortably and rest your left foot in your lap so that you can see the sole of your foot. Imagine a line dividing the sole in half horizontally. Be sure to measure from the tip of your big toe to the base of your heel and then divide this length in half.

Next, imagine a second line dividing your foot in half vertically. These two lines create four quadrants. On your left foot, the Kidney point is located primarily in the top left quadrant.

Place your thumb pad just above the horizontal line and to the left of the vertical line so that you're in the top left quadrant. To test this point, press firmly with your thumb. You can increase the pressure by leaning in with your body weight. You can also use the knuckle of your right index finger to press on the point. After pressing, slide your knuckle or thumb pad up slightly and press again. Continue until you are just below the ball of your foot.

Rate Your Sensitivity Level

Give your Kidney point an overall rating between 0 and 5 according to the following scale:

- **0:** The point is not sensitive at all. You can't feel a thing other than the sensation of pressing on your foot.

- **1:** It feels uncomfortable to press on the point. It's just below the threshold of what you would describe as pain.

- **2:** The point is quite sensitive with pressure, and you feel pain as you increase the pressure.

- **3:** The point hurts when you press on it. Definitely painful.

- **4:** The point is very painful and almost makes your eyes water when you press on it.

- **5:** @#%! It feels extremely painful even with light pressure.

What It Means When Your Kidney Point Is Sensitive

There are many reasons why your Kidney point may be sensitive. To understand the big picture, you need to view this in relation to your other reflexology points, overall constitution, and lifestyle.

For example, someone would have a sensitive Kidney point if they have or had kidney issues such as kidney stones or chronic kidney disease. They could also have a sensitive point if they've been taking medication for a long period of time because their kidneys have to work harder to filter the excess medication.

However, for the purpose of this exercise, we'll focus on what this point says about your life force energy levels.

Rating: 0 or 1

Ideally, if your qi is strong and robust, you would rate your sensitivity level as zero. I've only met one person who had a zero rating the first time I pressed on their Kidney point. He was a vegan college student and barefoot runner. Since he was jogging barefoot on rocky trails, it was like he was getting a foot reflexology session every time he went for a run. If you don't feel anything when you press on this point, and you're not a vegan barefoot runner, chances are you need to press harder.

A rating of one suggests that overall, you are very healthy, or your general constitution is very robust. You have excellent energy levels, but you may be doing a little too much lately. It would be good to relax and recharge.

Rating: 2 or 3

This suggests that you have been depleting your qi over time. Using the cell phone analogy, your battery is only half-charged. It is important that you stop pushing yourself or giving too much of your energy to others. It would be very beneficial for you to make time and space in your life for rest and rejuvenation and to nurture yourself.

Rating: 4 or 5

Your Kidney qi is weak and has been depleted over many years. It could be that you are a type A personality, pushing yourself too hard. Or if you're a type B, you've been putting the needs of others ahead of your own. This is your wake-up call that you really need to focus on resting and recharging. *You* should be your number one priority right now.

How to Boost Your Life Force

To replenish your life force, you have to eliminate what is draining your energy. Start at the root of the problem. I've observed that people with Kidney deficiencies tend to have similar characteristics. Ask yourself the following questions to see if this sounds like you:

1. Do you put the needs of other people ahead of your own? Do you give too much of yourself to others?

2. Are you an overachiever? Do you push yourself when you know you should be resting? Do you work too hard?

I understand that it's hard to change who you are. However, it is simple to make a small shift in your thinking or to change one choice you make today.

For example, if you're feeling tired, but think you "should" go for a run today, skip it. If you're thinking about working late to finish a report, turn off the computer a half hour earlier than you would normally. If someone asks you for a favor, today is the day you tell them, "No."

Every time you have a decision to make, choose the one that is most nurturing. It may go against all of your previous conditioning and habits, but over time you will see that by doing less, you actually get more done. When you recharge your batteries, you'll be more effective because you'll have abundant energy to invest in everything you do.

2. Chinese Reflexology Point for the Temporal Area

Use It to Check: Whether you have energy blocks in your head.

Why It Matters: The temporal point is a good indicator for how well qi is flowing to and from your head. Your temporal area is located on the side of your head at your temples, and also includes the area above and around your ears.

If your temporal point is sensitive, chances are that you hold a lot of tension in your neck, head, jaw, or face. Everything is interconnected, so when qi is not flowing smoothly to and from your head, it can lead to insufficient blood and nourishment flowing to these parts. It can also lead to a traffic jam of qi congesting in your head, and this can result in pain.

In Chinese Medicine, qi disruptions through the temporal area are associated with these conditions:

- Headaches and migraines
- Tinnitus (ringing in the ear), hearing loss
- Swelling and redness in the face
- TMJ, toothache, deviation of the mouth and jaw
- Stiff neck
- Dizziness

And this is just for the temporal area. Since this point is a general indicator of the flow of qi through your entire head, it can give you a heads-up (bad pun intended) on what's going on with your head.

I used to be a chronic overthinker, and as a result, I was disconnected from my heart and body. When I had my aura picture taken (it's a photo where your personal energy field shows up like a big cloud of color surrounding your body) at the psychic fair, the psychic would always comment that my energy was concentrated up in my head.

When I was in my 20s, this clustering of energy hadn't yet affected my health and well-being. As the years passed and the energy disharmony continued unchecked, however, it began to manifest in my body. I became very susceptible to insomnia because the concentration of qi in my head kept me awake at night.

While this particular qi disruption showed up as insomnia for me, it's different for everyone. But the solution is always the same: balance the flow of energy and eliminate the root cause of the disruption. That's what I did and as a result, I now sleep like a log!

How to Test Your Temporal Area Reflexology Point

The Chinese reflexology point for the temporal area of your head is located on the inside of your big toe. Before touching this point, first feel the pads of your toes. Notice how they feel relatively spongy and soft to touch.

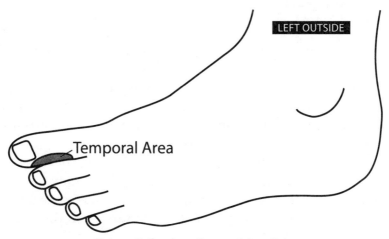

Chinese Reflexology Temporal Area Point

Then, use your thumb or index finger to press on the inside of the big toe on your left foot. Start at the tip of your toe and work your way down.

Rate Your Sensitivity Level

If you experience regular migraines or headaches, this point is likely to be sensitive. However, it is tricky to apply deep pressure on this point using your fingers, so it's quite likely that you won't feel too much in terms of sensitivity. What you want to be feeling for is how hard the inside of your toe feels to your touch:

- **Soft, supple, and spongy:** Qi is flowing smoothly if this area feels supple and spongy like your toe pad.

- **Hard, like the surface of a rock:** Qi is not flowing smoothly when this area feels hard to touch. Even if you're pressing on the bone, it would still feel a bit spongy on top if the qi was flowing smoothly. The harder this area feels, the greater the energy disruption.

How to Improve the Flow of Qi to Your Head

You can massage this point to help improve the flow of qi. You'll learn more on how to do this in an upcoming chapter. However, what is more important is to address the root cause of the energy disharmony, otherwise you'll simply be clearing energy and then it will block up again. It's like scooping water out of a boat with a hole in it. With enough scooping, you can empty the boat of water, but then it quickly fills up again until you fix the hole.

Here's what can disrupt the flow of qi to and from your head:

- Thinking too much, always analyzing things, being in your head

- Worrying

- Tension in your jaw, face, and neck

As a reformed overthinker, I have lots of experience with this. I also know that birds of a feather flock together, so you might not even realize the extent to which you're experiencing life in your head because most of the people around you seem just like you.

Here are a few telltale signs:

- You are not an overly emotional person and rarely express your feelings to others.

- Sometimes you think you should feel more, but you don't feel anything. It doesn't really concern you too much.

- You are very intelligent and like to analyze things.

- You work in a job that requires you to use your brain a lot.

- You are an excellent observer and tend to be introverted.

- You were a star academic student in school.

The problem with thinking too much is that it disconnects you from your body, heart, and soul. Your mind leads your life, and as a result, you approach everything this way. You research to solve your health problems because you've forgotten how to listen to your body. There is no better healer than your body, but you have to listen to it.

Here's one simple thing to start turning things around. For one day, choose from your heart and not your head: The next time you have a decision to make, don't make a list of pros and cons, don't poll your friends, and don't research online. Instead, choose impulsively, based on what *feels good* even if it makes no logical sense.

I have a theory that's why iPhones became so popular. When comparing price and functionality, the iPhones were more expensive than other options, but people enjoyed using them and liked the way they looked. If something makes you feel good, and it's not hurting anyone (including yourself), then choose it. Feeling good boosts your energy levels and helps your qi flow.

3. Chinese Reflexology Point for Lymphatic Drainage

Use It to Check: Whether you need to be more physically active.

Why It Matters: As a society, we are now realizing that too much sitting can negatively affect our health. Excessive sitting is being linked to heart attacks, cardiovascular disease, high blood pressure, and obesity.

So, what's considered "too much"? It's easy to find out from your body by checking your Chinese reflexology point for lymphatic drainage.

The lymphatic system plays a major role in supporting your immune system. It helps to distribute white blood cells throughout your body to fight infection, and it also helps clear waste and toxins. It's a lot like your circulatory system, only it circulates lymph fluid instead of blood.

Unlike your circulatory system, where your heart pumps blood throughout the body, there is no organ to pump lymph fluid. *It* moves when *you* move. Thus, if you don't get as much activity as your body needs, energy disharmonies will show up in your lymphatic system.

How to Test Your Lymphatic Drainage Reflexology Point

This reflexology point is located in the webbing between the bones of your big toe and second toe. To check this point, use the knuckle of your index finger. Press into the webbing at the base of your toes and then stroke downward toward the bottom of the V where the bones meet. Go slowly and press firmly.

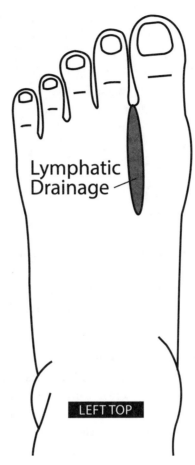

Chinese Reflexology Lymphatic Drainage Point

Rate Your Sensitivity Level

Give the point a rating between 0 and 5 using the scale you used for the Kidney reflexology point. Here's what the ratings tell you:

Rating: 0 or 1

If you rate this point as a zero, then qi and lymph are flowing smoothly through your body, and joy is flowing through your life.

However, in my experience, I have not encountered a single adult who did not have a sensitive lymphatic drainage point—not even the vegan barefoot runner.

Small children, on the other hand, normally don't feel a thing. I usually don't massage this point on kids because they're so active that they don't *need* this point massaged. The adults are another story! So if you're not feeling anything, press harder and also along the edge of the bones.

A rating of one suggests that you maintain a good level of activity throughout the day and you are generally a happy person. Keep it up!

Rating: 2 or 3

This suggests that you are probably sedentary for extended periods of time. It would be beneficial to exercise more and take breaks throughout the day to get up and move. In fact, stand up right now, stretch, and shake your body. Your qi will thank you.

Rating: 4 or 5

If this point is very sensitive, all of the above applies (for the rating of 2 or 3). Physical symptoms may be present such as tiredness, less resilience when it comes to fighting off colds, or swelling in the lymph nodes. If this is allowed to continue over time, it can lead to disorders related to poor functioning of the lymphatic system.

What if You Are Very Active and the Point Is Still Sensitive?

While this point can let you know if you need more physical activity, it can also tell you how much joy you are allowing to flow into your life. Thus, someone could be a marathon runner but still have a sensitive lymphatic drainage point because they cut themselves off from experiencing joy, and as a result, this constricts the flow of qi in their body.

How to Boost Your Lymphatic System

The true root of the problem isn't that someone is a couch potato, but that their lives could use more joy and passion. When you're not engaged in life, or when you feel unmotivated or stuck, you tend to procrastinate and avoid participating in life. These are indicators that you're not doing what lights your fire.

When I sit down to write an article for my blog, I'm usually doing it from a place of joy. As such, I find I naturally get up and move about quite regularly. However, there are times I am not writing from a place of joy. That's when I'm pushing myself to get an article finished because I have an imaginary deadline in my mind for writing a certain quota of articles each month. Then I realize I'm not writing from joy, and I remember to reconnect with the fun of creating and sharing.

When you're not choosing from joy, life often feels like a struggle, and you are doing a real disservice to your body. To turn things around, you certainly can get up and move more, but you also need to welcome more joy, fun, and play into your life. There must be something you really enjoyed doing as a child. Make it a priority to do it this week.

In addition, for the next 24 hours, be conscious of your choices. Are you choosing what you should be doing versus what you really want to do? Try choosing what feels most joyful. If you consistently do this over time, you will feel happier and more engaged in life. As a result, you'll feel more energized, and you will naturally move and be more active.

Now that you have a sense of where you are starting from, it's time to begin your joyful journey to heal your body and follow your bliss. It all begins with a single step, so let's move on to the first catalyst for healing your body: shifting the mind.

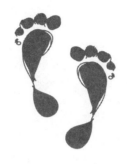

THE FIRST CATALYST

SHIFTING THE MIND
TO HEAL THE BODY

CHAPTER 3

Why Healing Begins with Your Mind

Your mind may be slowly killing you. Think not? If you *think* this isn't possible, your mind may already have you hoodwinked. To assess the damage, let's walk through a simple two-minute exercise that can reveal how much influence your mind really has on your health and well-being.

Have you ever been so upset over a situation that you kept replaying it in your mind for days afterward? Maybe you got pulled over for speeding even though you were going with the flow of traffic, and everyone else got away scot-free. Maybe a friend took advantage of your generosity multiple times, but failed to reciprocate the one time you asked her for help. Perhaps your boss overlooked you for a raise for the third year in a row.

Take a moment to think about a time when somebody did something or failed to do something, and it royally pissed you off. Go ahead and let yourself get good and angry. Think back to the scene or situation—really place yourself there as you were experiencing it. Who was involved?

Replay the scenario in your head. Hear the words that were said or the words that were not said, but should have been. Direct all your anger at the one person or group of people that made you hopping mad. Then—

Sorry to interrupt your thoughts here, but did you happen to notice what was going on in your body as you recalled this memory? Did you notice tension in your body? Where were you feeling it? Go through the following list and note where you hold stress in your body.

- Jaw
- Neck
- Shoulders
- Hands
- Stomach
- Other?
- All of the above!

While you're at it, did you also notice your breathing? You may have been holding your breath or breathing more rapidly. What about your heart rate? Was your heart beating just a little bit faster?

Now that you've observed the effect of anger on your body, let's move on to the next part of this exercise. Think of a really sad time in your life. It may have been triggered by the loss of a beloved pet, the ending of a relationship, or the death of a close family member. Whatever it was, go back to the memory and really immerse yourself in that time and space. What thoughts were going through your head?

Was it a sudden shock or was it something you could see coming? Who was there with you, or were you alone in your grief? For the purpose of this exercise, allow yourself to be in the depths of your thoughts and feelings for about 10 to 15 seconds.

Pay attention to where you're feeling the sadness in your body. Is there a hollow ache in your chest? Is there a pain in your heart? Are you suddenly taking shallow breaths? Do you feel like curling up into a ball?

Okay, that's enough of the negative feelings. It's time to visit a happy place. Think of a time in your life when you felt incredible joy. It may have been when you were a child. It may have been the birth of a child. Perhaps you were traveling and experienced a sense of freedom, exploration, and adventure. Maybe it was when you found your soul mate.

Similar to how you allowed yourself to dive fully into a sad memory, give yourself the gift of being fully present in this moment of joy. What was making you feel so happy? Who was there? Experience it again in your mind's eye, and revel in your happiness for at least a minute.

Now notice what's going on in your body. Is there a feeling of warmth surrounding your heart? Do you feel relaxed and energized at the same time? You've probably taken a few deep breaths, and your lips may have turned up in a smile.

From this simple exercise of recalling three different memories, you can see that thoughts and feelings can evoke different physical reactions. You can create stress in your body simply by what you choose to think about.

Nothing has changed from the beginning of this chapter to the point where you are reading now. You are still sitting where you were five minutes ago. Everything stayed exactly the same with one exception—where you were directing your thoughts.

When you are recalling an emotion, whether it is anger, sadness, or joy, you're probably not thinking too much because you are feeling. However, it's your mind that replays a memory over and over again as if it were an interactive movie. It's your mind that keeps track of the story and the characters. And it's your mind that chooses to buy a ticket to one movie over another.

Do you really want to watch *Sad Times of My Life,* or *I Am Seriously Pissed at You Part XXXIV* for days on end? I saw *Mortal Kombat* (yes, the movie based on the '90s video game) in the theater five times, but that was when I was young and foolish. Those were the years before I had a kid and could squander my time away. The movie was fun and kitschy, but admittedly, it lost the initial luster after multiple viewings.

The same holds true for thoughts and memories that replay in your head. Your mind loves to analyze things to death, and what better fodder to examine than the episodes of your life? And just like in the movies, it's the tension and drama that draws in the viewers.

Replaying thoughts and memories is so natural that we often don't realize how much we do it. You've probably heard the figure floating around on the Internet that the average person has 60,000 thoughts per day, and 95 percent of these are the same thoughts as the day before.

Whether or not this is true for you, these numbers can inspire you to pause and evaluate how often you repeat the same thoughts in your head. It's probably a lot more than you think. The problem with thinking the same things over and over again is that it's easy for your mind to get stuck, as we'll soon get into. Next thing you know, you're in your head all the time, and your mind has taken control of your life.

Constantly thinking, analyzing, worrying, and replaying the past in your head takes you away from the present moment. It takes you away from your awareness of the here and now. When you're disconnected from the present moment, you are also disconnected from your body, heart, and soul. You cut yourself off from the voice that knows what you need to heal and thrive, the important connection to your inner guidance.

Aside from the observable effects on your body, being stuck in your head has an even more insidious effect on your physical health. In the earlier exercise, you saw how your thoughts could create tension in your body and change your breathing and heart rate. Those same thoughts are also seriously affecting something else that you're probably not even aware of.

Your Thoughts Can Disrupt the Flow of Qi

When you are experiencing stress and negative emotions, there is tension not only at the physical level but also at the energy level. The tension in your muscles and tendons obstructs the smooth flow of qi throughout your body. It's similar to how a tight elastic band would cut off the flow of blood through your veins—only instead of an elastic, it's the tension in your body that is cutting off the flow of qi.

Fortunately, the effects are usually temporary and dissipate when you let go of the negative thoughts and emotions and simply relax. That's because qi always wants to flow as it should, and it wants to be in balance.

However, if you hold on to the negativity, you never fully release the tension in your body. Thus, the cumulative effects of where you direct your thoughts over the course of the days, weeks, months, and years of your life eventually alters the flow of qi in your body—depleting the flow in some areas, or causing it to become blocked in others.

It's easy to understand this connection when you compare the flow of qi to a river. When the river is flowing smoothly, then the ecosystem is in balance. The same holds true for your body. If a negative thought crosses your mind, it's like tossing a twig into a flowing river: While it may cause a slight ripple or a temporary disruption to the flow of qi, the current eventually carries it away.

However, if you are constantly tossing twigs and debris into the river, the water gets murky and the river becomes less efficient at clearing things away. Eventually, the river gets plugged up, and this leads to problems both upstream and downstream. The banks overflow before the obstruction, and the downstream riverbed dries out.

Just like the river, an energy obstruction in your body could result in too much qi in one area and a lack of qi in another. When qi is flowing as it should, your body is well. That's because qi is the life force energy that powers your body's systems—it helps everything run smoothly and efficiently. When qi is not in balance, your body can get out of balance, and this is when *dis-ease* moves from the energy level to the physical level.

While the flow of qi is altered by your thoughts, it is also impacted by your actions or inaction. And guess who's in charge of that? Yup, your mind.

Have you ever done something that you didn't want to, but you did it because you had to do it or you thought you *should* do it? Did you notice how exhausted you felt afterward? It was totally qi depleting.

The root of most health problems is allowing the mind to direct your life. It guides you into fear, stress, struggle, and judgment. It makes you do things that you don't want to that drain your life force energy. And most significantly, your mind disconnects you from your body, heart, and soul so that you can no longer hear your inner guidance.

So how do you begin to turn things around? Well, just as your mind has the power to disrupt the flow of qi, it also can be used to *harmonize* the qi in your body. While you just saw a few minutes ago how your thoughts and feelings can negatively impact your body, you also witnessed how a joyful memory and happy thoughts made you feel good.

One of the most powerful catalysts for health and vitality is to shift your mind to heal your body. If your mind got you into this mess, it can get you out of it, too. While your mind may be a tenacious and stubborn partner, it's not evil or malicious. Your mind wants you to be well. That's *why* it loves to analyze and replay memories. It's trying to find a solution to your problems. It's also trying to create a sense of control by keeping things the same. You just have to show it that change is going to lead to something better. It takes a little bit of convincing, but it is possible.

First you have to understand *why* your mind thinks that being in control is what's best for you. I actually stumbled upon this answer by accident.

Your Mind Wants to Protect You

When I first began doing Dragon Spirit work with clients, I noticed a pattern emerge. Every overthinker had one thing in common—an unusually traumatic childhood such as physical or emotional abuse, an alcoholic or mentally ill parent, or the breakup of the family.

If you met these people, you would never know that they held a dark secret inside. They were highly intelligent, well-spoken, and successful in their chosen career paths. From the outside looking in, my clients were the epitome of well-adjusted contributing members of society.

I remember when I first noticed the pattern, I thought, *How is it possible that so many of my clients have alcoholic parents? Does everyone have a parent with a drinking problem?*

It was definitely an *aha* moment when I realized that all of these people, who had struggled for years to figure out their life purpose, were blocked by their well-intentioned minds. Due to the trauma and lack of control they experienced as children, they had shut off their feelings and gone into their heads to survive.

Regardless of what the trauma was, there was always one defining moment in their childhood when their mind made a conscious decision to take charge because it gave them a sense of control and safety where they had none. It's interesting to note that even though their minds made the decision, the memory of the choice was usually buried deep within, and my clients had no conscious awareness of it—at least not until their Dragon Spirit session!

One client made this decision at her eighth birthday party. Aubrey had invited her friends over to her house for what was supposed to be a fun celebration. Midway through the party, her father barged into the room, drunk and belligerent. He criticized and humiliated her in front of her friends. Aubrey felt denigrated and ashamed. Her way of coping was to shut off her feelings and start choosing with her head instead of her heart. After all, if an open heart could lead to such pain, then it was better to ignore her heart. Aubrey stopped listening to her feelings and intuition, and as a result, she couldn't hear the calling of her soul to follow her life purpose.

Another client was riding her bike when she had a major wipe-out in front of her home. As Margaret lay on the sidewalk bleeding, no one came to her assistance. Margaret's mother suffered from mental illness, and as a result, was not the best of mothers. All the years of having an absent mom hit home, and this pain was much worse than the physical pain that Margaret was experiencing. She couldn't control her mother's disease, so she did the next best thing, which was to use her mind to control her feelings and her life.

When you're feeling helpless, shutting off your emotions and going into your head is a coping mechanism. Heck, people still do this as adults. How many times have you exercised control to stop yourself from crying in front of others? So you can imagine what it must be like for a small child. When you're a kid, you feel pretty small and helpless, so you do the best you can with what you have; and if that means letting your mind take charge, then so be it.

As an adult, however, this becomes a problem because the mind *continues* to protect you by trying to control your life. Even though you are much stronger and wiser than when you were a little kid, the pattern from childhood persists because it has become your default modus operandi. Out of *habit*, your mind acts as the gatekeeper of change, and the running monologue in your head is so loud that it drowns out your inner voice of wisdom.

So, what's your story? What happened to you when you were a child? Are you aware of it, or is it buried deep down inside? It's okay if you don't want to answer this question right now. And while you may not have had a traumatic childhood like some of my clients, we *all* have had moments where we felt hurt and vulnerable as young children. While we may conveniently forget these moments, our reactions to these emotions still influence our behavior today.

Sometimes the pain is hidden so deep within that you're not even consciously aware of it. For many of my clients, this was the case. After all, your mind is extremely clever. If you were a private investigator and your mind was a fugitive trying to elude the law, I would put my money on your mind. Fortunately, there are ways to outsmart it.

How to Shift the Mind to Heal Your Body

There are three steps to shift the mind for healing:

1. Awareness

2. Letting go

3. Believing you can heal and choosing to heal

These steps are much easier than your mind would lead you to believe. In fact, you've already completed the first step. Awareness is simply acknowledging that something in your life is not supporting your health and vitality.

In the previous chapter, you massaged three different Chinese reflexology points on your feet. The sensitivity of these points gave you an awareness of potential problem areas in your body and your life where you may be constricting the flow of qi. There wasn't any analyzing or second-guessing. Your feet very clearly told you whether or not your qi was flowing as it should.

In this chapter, you walked through a simple exercise recalling different memories from your life. You relived anger, sadness, and happiness, and observed how the corresponding thoughts and feelings affected your body.

Now that you have this awareness and understanding, you can start turning things around and using your mind to help you heal.

Congratulations! You're on your way, and you may not have even realized it. Let's keep going!

CHAPTER 4

LETTING GO

To keep up your forward momentum, let's deal with one of the biggest obstacles to healing your body, which is *letting go.* For optimal health—and a happy life—you must release any attachment you may have to the disease, ailment, or injury in your body. You also need to let go of any negative thoughts and feelings you have about your health.

It's difficult to welcome health and vitality with ease and flow if you are holding on to the thoughts and feelings that caused you to make the choices that created your current state of health. But when you let go of thoughts, feelings, and habits that no longer serve you, this clears the way to welcome ideas and actions that support your health and well-being.

Do you ever think, *I need my coffee to make it through the day,* or *I'm blind as a bat and can't see a thing without my glasses?* Your body hears your thoughts, and over time, it becomes what you think. Scarily, we are seldom aware of just how often we criticize our own bodies.

I had one client with a very sensitive reflexology point on the side of her foot. When I told her it was the Chinese reflexology point for her knee, she started telling me about her "bum knee" and how it bothered her so much that she wanted to "just cut it right off."

How can a knee heal when such venom is directed at it every day? It was like her knee was being bullied by the mean girls in high school. Don't let yourself be the mean girl to your own body!

Another woman I met at a party told me about her detached retina. We were having a perfectly normal party conversation when, out of nowhere, the story of her detached retina came up. When I suggested to her that it was possible to heal, she told me all the reasons why she had the problem, all the limitations she had as a result, and why she had accepted this was her lot in life. Quite frankly, she was rather attached to her detached retina.

Why We Have Attachment Issues

Logically speaking, you would think that no one would ever want to hold on to disease or discomfort. Nobody wants to be sick. Everybody wants to be healthy, right? If only we were that logical, then everyone would be in a perfect state of health. Unfortunately, there's a little glitch with our internal programming.

There are two reasons why you may be attached to a disease or ailment. The first is that your mind does not like change, and it tries to keep everything the same in order to protect you. When everything is stable, it gives you an illusion of control over your life, as we discussed in the previous chapter.

When you've had a health issue for a long time, it can become a part of your identity, which was the case for the woman with the detached retina. She introduced herself at a party and within minutes was talking about her eye problems.

The challenges she faced because of her eye condition played a significant role in shaping who she was as a person. This made her detached retina a part of her identity. If she were to completely heal her detached retina, she would shake the foundation of her self-identity, and this can be a very scary thing for the mind.

You may also be attached to a health condition because you get something from holding on to it—or at least your mind thinks you're better off because of it. The disease or ailment often gives you something that you are unwilling to give yourself.

For me, the example that immediately comes to mind is the car accident I was in. My family and I were on our way to my grandparents' wedding anniversary banquet dinner when we were sideswiped by another vehicle. We were in a tiny Honda Civic hatchback. The car that drove into us was a late '80s Mercedes. Those cars were enormous and built like tanks.

The brunt of the force hit the rear passenger on the driver's side of the car, who happened to be me. As a result, I had lateral whiplash and experienced chronic pain in my neck and shoulders for years after the accident. Interestingly, I would go through periods where I felt perfectly fine, but then do something innocuous, like reaching for a towel, that would trigger a pain episode that would last for days.

Who would want that in their life, right?

But I received a benefit from the accident. I was even conscious of it in the early days after being injured. In fact, I was excited by it. I loved it. That's why it took me such a long time to let it go.

The benefit I received from the car accident was the power to say, "No." Being in excruciating pain was the only way I could give myself permission to say no to everyone in my life who was making demands of me.

I remember that before the accident, I felt like I was being pulled in every direction. I was juggling the demands at the office where we were short-staffed, a new boyfriend who wanted to see me all the time, helping my mom look after a stray cat that had litter-box issues, dealing with my roommate who did not like the cat and was allergic to it, and trying to find time to spend with family and friends. Whew, my head's spinning just writing all of that.

On top of everything, I was also a karate fanatic at the time. I commuted over an hour each way for my karate class three times a week. At the time of the accident, I was two weeks away from testing for my blue belt, so I had increased the intensity and frequency of my training.

After the accident, I was in so much pain that I couldn't do anything. The benefit I received from holding on to the injury was that it gave me an excuse to say no. When I finally learned to say no, without using the accident as a crutch, that was when my body healed at a deeper level, and I let go of the chronic pain.

How to Let Go of Attachment

One of the easiest ways to let go of a disease or ailment is to identify the benefit you receive from it and then give that benefit to yourself. Until you do this, your mind will find it challenging to let go because it would appear that the disease or ailment is serving you. As a result, you may find yourself sabotaging your own healing without even realizing it.

Have you ever noticed how people struggle with yo-yo dieting? After losing weight, they find themselves gaining it back and then the pattern repeats. At an emotional level, weight is often viewed as a layer of protection. If being overweight gives someone a feeling of safety, it doesn't make any sense to lose the weight because that's like lowering the shields on the *Starship Enterprise*.

However, if the person finds other ways to create a feeling of security, such as boosting their confidence or releasing the fears that made them feel unsafe, then it is much easier for the mind to jump on board with a new direction.

Sometimes it may be hard to identify what your benefit is. You may see the pain, suffering, or inconvenience of a disease or ailment, but you're really left scratching your head trying to figure out how any of it is of benefit to you.

You can, however, get the answers you seek by moving beyond your logical mind and listening to your body. That's because disease or discomfort is your body's way of communicating a message from your heart and soul that you've been ignoring for a long time. Your body wants you to listen and is thrilled when you do.

One of my students, April, had a pain in the middle of her back for decades. It had been a part of April's body for so long that she never considered that she could ever be free of the pain. During her Dragon Spirit session, it was revealed that the pain first began when she was working at a factory. The work was hard and caused a lot of strain and fatigue in her shoulders, arms, and back. However, April loved her job because of the friendships she had with her co-workers.

They were a tight-knit group of women who enjoyed socializing together. The benefit that April received from holding on to the pain was that it reminded her of the camaraderie and close friendships. Letting go of the pain would have been like letting go of the good times and good friends.

In her present life, April was in the habit of prioritizing her family over "girlfriend time." She found it challenging to find time to spend with her friends because she was so busy caring for her family. What April really wanted was the same sense of sisterhood and fun that she had when she worked at the factory.

During her session, April identified ways she could create this in her life, including calling her friends more often and making the time to do this by watching less television. She made a commitment to start right away, and made it a priority to find time to nurture the relationships and connections that her heart was craving.

I heard from April about a month later. She told me that she had been following through on her commitment, and that her back was feeling better than ever. This was amazing to hear because she had been living with the back pain for decades. It had become so prevalent and pervasive that it was like background noise, and she had accepted that it would be with her for the rest of her life. However, within a few weeks of feeling more connected with her friends, she was already seeing an improvement.

All it takes is a small shift in direction—one degree—to alter the course of your health and transform your life. Changing your course by one degree doesn't make much difference when you walk a few feet, but if you think of the difference one degree makes to a boat's or plane's destination, you realize what a big impact it can have. What if the *Apollo 11* had been off by one degree on its trip to the moon?

So let's shift one degree right now by determining the benefit you receive from an ailment or health condition. The following Transform Your Attachment exercise will help you identify what your benefit is, and what you can do to start enriching your life right away.

How to Transform Your Attachment

While you might have something specific that you'd like to examine, it's best to tune in to your body and listen to its wisdom. For example, if you suffer from back pain, you may think that this is where you'd like to focus your attention. However, your body may wish to guide you in an entirely different direction. Maybe it wants you to let go of the blister on your foot first. And while this may seem completely unrelated to your back pain, you may need to let go of the blister before you can release the pain in your back.

When you approach healing from the perspective of finding a solution for a specific disease or ailment, you are coming at it from the mind's eye. Trust your body's innate wisdom. It wants you to be healthy, strong, free, flexible, and full of vitality. However, it may have a different path from what you have in mind.

In order to hear what your body wants you to let go of, I'll walk you through the Transform Your Attachment exercise.

Transform Your Attachment Exercise

You'll need about 10 to 15 minutes of quiet time to complete the exercise. So make sure you're comfy and have a block of distraction-free time. No texting, surfing the Internet, or watching TV at the same time. Give yourself the gift of being present. It's kind of neat how the word *present* also means gift.

To complete this exercise, you'll answer six questions. Begin by setting the intention to *listen to your body* for the answers, especially for the first four questions. Focus on what you're *feeling*, and this will help you hear what your body has to say. Your mind will get the opportunity to jump into the fray for the last two questions.

1. Where are you feeling *it* in your body?

It can best be described as a feeling or sensation in your body that attracts your attention. Don't *think* too much about *it* right now because thinking can distract you from hearing your body. So read through the instructions for this first question and then give it a go.

Begin by sitting quietly and focusing on your breathing for three to five minutes. I know that this can seem like an eternity if you're not used to meditating, but give it a try and do the best you can. And if you do meditate regularly, this may seem like child's play or scratching the surface. Set aside all thought and preconceived notions. (*Psst,* that's your mind talking.)

After sitting quietly for a few minutes, bring your awareness and attention to your body. Where do you feel something in your body? It may feel like an ache, discomfort, or pain. It could also feel like a tingle or a sense of warmth. If you notice your attention being drawn to more than one area in your body, take note of what caught your attention first.

2. What does this feeling represent?

Once you've identified where *it* is in your body that's calling your attention, bring all of your awareness to that area. Focus your energy there and ask yourself, "What does this represent?"

How your body answers this question will be different for everyone. Some people feel a physical sensation while others may have words, images, or memories come to mind. Allow whatever comes through to flow without judgment, even if it seems like it can't be right or if it feels like a really bad cliché. If nothing comes to mind, give yourself permission to use your imagination and just go with it.

When I guided a group of students through this exercise in my online program, I answered the questions for myself along with them. Where I first noticed a feeling in my body was in my shoulders. It felt like a sense of tightness. As I brought my full attention, energy, and awareness to my shoulders, the answer I received came in the form of four words, which were *weight of the world.*

3. What benefit do you get from having this?

After answering question number two, continue paying attention to this area of your body as you ask yourself, "What benefit do I get from having this?"

The answer may come as a whisper that makes you question whether it was real, or it may come as a loud voice shouting inside your mind. And if you hear nothing, allow yourself to use your imagination. Pretend that you're getting a message and see what it is.

While I was doing this exercise with my students, the answer I received wasn't all that flattering. These answers often aren't easy on the ego. For me, the weight of the world gave me the benefit of a sense of importance. It made me feel like I mattered because I was supporting the world.

4. What is the gift that you really want?

Ask your body, "What can I give myself instead of holding on to this?" Allow whatever pops into your mind to be the answer. *Do not overthink this!* If you find yourself getting caught up in your head, return your focus to where you experienced the feeling of *it* in your body.

For me, what came to mind was that I desired a feeling of importance because I wasn't appreciating myself enough—specifically, I was not appreciating my value and my accomplishments.

Being Asian, it's very uncouth to brag. You keep your successes to yourself, and you always minimize them as if anybody could have done what you did, but you were just lucky. Chinese parents do this all the time. For example, they might say, "My son goes to Stanford, but he only got accepted because the applicant pool was very weak that year. Besides, Stanford is for the kids who are not bright enough to get into Harvard."

Growing up with these cultural norms, I downplayed everything I accomplished, no matter how extraordinary it was. The gift I wanted to give myself was to feel okay with being exceptional and not have to hide it. Instead of minimizing my achievements, I wanted to own them. I was longing for a sense of importance because I was not making myself feel important and not valuing what I had accomplished.

5. What does this look like?

Now it's time for your mind to shine because you're going to direct its analytical powers to make a very important list. You're going to *think* of all the tangible actions that you could take to give yourself the gift that you really want. So bust out a pen and paper and write down your list.

The actions should be things that you can picture yourself doing as if you were watching a movie of your life. The reason it should be something that you can visualize is because when you are *doing* the action, it helps get you out of your head. Even if you wrote *meditating* on your list, you could still envision yourself sitting in a meditative posture during a quiet moment in the morning. Seeing yourself doing the activity helps you create the time and space to make it happen.

6. What do you focus on now?

After you've made your list, choose one of the items to do today. While it may not immediately give you the gift you seek, once you begin, you will get more ideas on how to follow through so that you can give yourself the benefit that you need.

My first action was to appreciate my accomplishments by sharing one of them on Facebook. I found the postcards I had sent to myself during my cross-Canada bicycle trip. For years, they'd been hidden in a plastic bag in a memento box shoved in a corner of the bedroom closet.

I took pictures of every postcard from British Columbia to Ontario and shared the photos online. I told my friends that I had ridden a bicycle across Canada. Dang, that was pretty awesome of me!

Eventually, that first action led to other actions where I became more and more appreciative of my value and accomplishments. This gave me an insane level of confidence and gutsiness that opened up numerous opportunities for me to share Chinese reflexology to even bigger audiences than before.

Now that you've gone through the Transform Your Attachment exercise, I will let you in on a little secret. Remember when I told you to pretend you were getting a message if nothing came to mind? That was a clever trick to stop your mind from acting as a gatekeeper and blocking the messages from your body, heart, and soul. If your mind thinks you're only pretending, you can sneak the messages through.

Before you read any further, review your answer to question six of the exercise. Have you completed that action yet? If not, stop and do it right now. If you can't work on it immediately, then write down a *specific* time and date (preferably today) for when you'll complete it.

The sooner you start, the sooner your body knows that you heard the message loud and clear, and it can stop using the disease or discomfort to draw your attention. And when you start giving yourself the benefit that you seek, you break free of past patterns and start creating momentum toward amazing health and vitality. You can let go of anything—even if you've held on to it for years.

Shortly after I started valuing myself, I enrolled in a karate class. I had practiced martial arts for years up until the car accident. During the years following the accident, I periodically tried to return to martial arts, but it was always too hard on my body—especially my neck and shoulders. I ended up letting go of martial arts even though I had enjoyed it so much.

As I discovered the catalysts for healing and applied them to my life, I released 99.99 percent of the accident from my body. The last frontier was to return to martial arts. Appreciating my value was what I needed to do in order to let go of the last 0.01 percent of residual energy held in my shoulders.

After my first karate class, I was sore and aching all over, but my shoulders held up just fine. In fact, by the third week, it was getting easy to do full push-ups. (*Shh,* don't tell anyone, or I'll never be able to slack off in the back row again!)

CHAPTER 5

BELIEVING AND CHOOSING HEALTH

If you want to heal your body, you've got to choose to heal. But before you can do that, you have to *believe* you can heal. If you doubt yourself, you'll limit the extent of your healing to what you consciously or subconsciously believe is possible.

Belief is the magic ingredient for taking inspired action toward your goals. Think about it—would you take action if you thought you were going to fail? If there was no chance for success, you wouldn't bother. And that's what stops most people. It is not that they're lazy, stupid, or manifesting the wrong way. It's because they're missing the key element linking thought to action, which is belief.

Believing You Deserve Health and Vitality

In addition to believing that healing is possible, you also have to believe that you *deserve* to heal. Guilt is a powerful emotion that can hold us back because we punish ourselves for something we did or didn't do in the past. Holding guilt inside our bodies creates an energetic block, which disrupts the flow of qi.

Such was the case for Jeannette. Although she had always been strong and healthy, she had recently developed a very painful medical condition related to her reproductive system.

Jeannette shared that she had cheated on her boyfriend in the past. While she had ended the affair and had refocused her energies on repairing her relationship, she was wracked with guilt. She held all of the guilt inside her reproductive system. What better way to internalize her guilt than to hold it in her sexual organs?

Her guilt was so strong that she believed she deserved to suffer, and she concentrated all of her negative emotions in the area "responsible" for her affair. The resulting disruption to the flow of qi was so strong that the energetic block quickly transformed into a physical problem.

Jeannette was consciously aware that her health condition was related to the affair. Because she already knew the emotional root of her ailment, we focused her Dragon Spirit session on helping her find a path for self-forgiveness.

When I guided her to hear her inner wisdom—without the interference or judgment of her mind, she recognized the strong soul connection between herself and the man she had an affair with. Her soul let her know that she was not a "bad" person, but that what had drawn the two of them together was simply the many past lives they had shared together. Interestingly, she also discovered that she had shared many past lives with her boyfriend, too.

When Jeannette saw how their three souls had been intertwined for many lifetimes, she was able to begin the process of forgiving herself. She began to let go of the belief that she deserved to be punished. She had already suffered enough. It was time to let go and move forward.

When she started to believe she deserved to get better, her body responded very quickly. Within several weeks, there was a dramatic improvement in her condition, and she was on her way to returning to robust health.

If you're holding on to guilt, it is so important to forgive yourself. You *are* deserving of health and vitality, and we're planting the seed right now so that you can start the process of forgiveness.

Begin with 0.01 Percent Belief

The good news is that you don't have to believe 100 percent in your ability to heal, or fully embrace that you're deserving of amazing health and vitality. If everyone waited until they were 100 percent sure of something, not a whole lot would get done. Instead, you only have to start with 0.01 percent belief in what you're capable of accomplishing—and that you *deserve* it. Nurture this belief like a seed, and when you do, it will sprout up like a magic beanstalk.

First, you have to know what you want. After all, you can't believe something is possible if you have no idea what that something is. What does your image of health and vitality look like? What do you want to release from your body? How do you want to feel when you wake up every morning?

As long as you have a general idea of where you're heading, it doesn't matter what your goal is—whether you see it as small and inconsequential or so big that it feels almost impossible. What matters is that you have a destination in mind because that will send you in the right direction. And as your health improves, you'll also change your vision of what you believe is possible.

For example, someone who has a migraine may initially decide that their vision of health is to get immediate pain relief. Once the pain is gone, they'll then want to reduce the number of headaches they get each month. When that starts happening, their idea of health will shift from not getting migraines to improving their overall health.

Visualize Where You Want Your Health to Be

Visualization is a powerful tool for creating a clear picture of where you want to be in terms of your health and well-being. If you can recall a childhood memory or imagine yourself sitting on a beach, then you have all the tools you need to visualize health and vitality.

Visualization can also be used to activate the muscle memory of health in your body. If you've ever mastered a physical activity, such as riding a bicycle or playing a musical instrument, you know that after many hours of practice, you reach a point where you don't have to think about what you're doing anymore because your body is acting on autopilot. That's muscle memory. Even if you haven't been on a bicycle in years, your body remembers how—"it's just like riding a bike!"

I experienced the power of muscle memory quite dramatically when I went to my first karate class after almost two decades of not training. Even though I hadn't practiced in years, I was able to follow along in class quite easily. I couldn't remember much with my brain, but my body remembered how to move.

To activate the muscle memory of health, all you need to do is remember when you were healthy. Perhaps there's a memory from childhood or college days when you felt young and free without the constraints, judgments, and emotional baggage that we tend to pick up through the years. Back then, you didn't beat yourself up over things that you should or shouldn't have done. And remember when you didn't worry about your weight, food sensitivities, stress levels, or that pain in your lower back because everything in your body was working exactly as it should.

Hold that vision in your mind's eye. Experience the feeling of strength, energy, and vitality in your body. Feel the lightness of your emotions. This can be your vision of where you want to return.

Another visualization technique is to activate a future memory of health. Since you haven't lived it yet, you don't have a real memory to draw upon, but you can use your imagination. If you can imagine yourself going on vacation, then you can imagine yourself in optimal health.

Picture yourself doing something that you have always wanted to do that requires your body to be strong and healthy. Since you're imagining, give yourself permission to visualize without any constraints. For example, if you want to climb Mount Fuji, don't worry about how you're going to get to Japan, what gear you may need, or even how you'll overcome a fear of heights. Instead, make it a given that you have everything you need to climb Mount Fuji. Imagine yourself hiking the trails, breathing in the air, and feeling alive and full of energy.

Go ahead and take a minute or two to visualize yourself on an adventure. Really revel in the experience. See yourself there and feel your excitement. Your sense of adventure helps to keep negative emotions such as guilt and worry at bay. Breathe in deeply as you feel your body going through the motions of the activity. Hear it, smell it, and taste it if you can. After you have imagined it, you have opened the door of possibility by 0.01 percent.

Stepping-stone Affirmations

Once you have your vision in mind, all you need to do is keep moving the needle of your belief until the vision becomes your reality. Start with a 0.01 percent possibility, and when that feels good for you, move on to 0.02 percent. By shifting your belief in tiny increments over time, you expand your belief in what is possible.

You also release the stranglehold that *disbelief* has on the flow of qi in your body. When your thoughts are rigid, you can almost visualize what that looks like in your body: rigid, inflexible, unmoving—everything that is the exact opposite of what qi should be, which is flowing.

When you reach beyond your current way of thinking, you increase the likelihood of finding what will help your body heal. In addition, when your belief grows, you are more likely to follow through with activities and thoughts that support your health and vitality. I experienced this myself firsthand after my car accident. I had to let go of my rigid beliefs about pain and start believing I could heal my body *before* I could find the things that helped me heal.

To expand your thinking, you have to say good-bye to limiting beliefs and negative emotions that hold you back and make you doubt your ability to succeed. People often use affirmations to help reprogram their thoughts by repeating positive statements to themselves.

However, affirmations don't always work for everyone. Admittedly, I used to think affirmations were useless, and I'd roll my eyes whenever someone mentioned them. It's not that I didn't try to use affirmations—I really did try wholeheartedly, but they didn't seem to work for me.

I've stood in front of a mirror and repeated nice frilly sentences to myself. I've followed other people's advice to touch my elbows to my knees while proclaiming with over-the-top enthusiasm a top ten list of affirmations. I've bellowed at full volume, only to drift off when I glanced at the piece of paper to read what I was affirming. After a few weeks of doing this, I'd look at my life and see that nothing had changed.

That's what affirmations were like for me until I realized what the problem was. Once I made a few tweaks, affirmations that had me rolling my eyes before were rolling off my tongue smoother than a cheesy compliment from a pickup artist. More importantly, they started working!

If you've found in the past that affirmations don't work for you, it may be because your mind has been working against you. That was what happened to me. When you have an analytical brain, saying affirmations can actually hinder your progress. That's because every time you say or think an affirmation, your mind takes stock of your current situation and sees that your reality is different from what you are affirming. Your mind is like a private investigator catching a witness in a lie. Every time you say the affirmation, your mind exclaims, *That's not true!*

As a result, instead of affirming what you want to happen, you are affirming the opposite. For example, if you feel sick and tired and say the affirmation "I feel energized and healthy," your mind observes that you actually feel sick and tired. Thus, every time you repeat the positive affirmation, your mind thinks, *I'm not really feeling that.* So, it's affirming that the affirmation is not true.

Instead of making an affirmation that contradicts your observed reality, you have to start with a statement that your mind can accept as true. Then, you continue your progress by using what I call *stepping-stone affirmations.* Each stepping-stone nudges you along a continuum of belief until you totally believe the positive affirmation. The stones are like a path leading you up the mountain until you reach the summit of Mount Fuji.

For your first stepping-stone, I suggest starting with the phrase, "It is not entirely impossible." This phrase is open-ended enough that almost anything that follows it could be true. For example, I could say it is not entirely impossible that I could win the lottery. This would be a true statement because if I am able to buy a ticket, then it's not entirely impossible that I could win.

Stepping-stone Affirmations for Healing

Here are sample stepping-stone affirmations for health and vitality. They can take you from whatever state your health is in right now to the strong belief "I am healing my body."

1. *It is not entirely impossible* that I could heal my body.

2. *It is not impossible* that I could heal my body.

3. *There is a very small chance, but it is not impossible* that I could heal my body.

4. *While it's highly unlikely, it is possible* that I could heal my body.

5. *While I don't fully believe it, it is possible* that I could heal my body.

6. *There is a possibility* that I could heal my body.

7. *It is possible* that I could heal my body.

8. *I could* heal my body.

9. *I can* heal my body.

10. *I am* healing my body.

Take a minute to come up with your own stepping-stone affirmation right now. Begin with the phrase "It is not entirely impossible," and then use your own words to complete the sentence. I find that repeating affirmations in my own words is much more powerful than using someone else's words, so feel free to use these sample stepping-stone affirmations as a guide, and modify them however you'd like.

Repeat your first stepping-stone affirmation out loud. How does it feel? Is it believable? Adjust the wording until it feels like a credible statement. Repeat it occasionally throughout the day until it rings true for you. Once it does, move on to your next stepping-stone affirmation, and continue progressing at a pace that feels right for you. It may take minutes, days, weeks, or even months before you truly believe an affirmation, but don't worry about the timeline.

Progress is not measured by how fast you move through your list of stepping-stone affirmations. The secret to progress is to *not* measure your progress. All you have to do is feel good that you're doing something positive for yourself. That's it.

How to Really Get Your Qi Flowing

On the path to ascend your metaphoric Mount Fuji, one of the biggest obstacles you'll encounter is negative emotions. You've already learned how emotions can evoke tension in your body and adversely affect the flow of qi. These emotions can also *stop* you from believing.

If you want to free your qi and power up your affirmation stepping-stones, the best way to do this is to raise your energetic vibration. Every living thing is comprised of energy—*you* are comprised of energy, and your life force has an energetic vibration. In babies, this frequency is naturally high, but by adulthood it gets bogged down with poor choices, lack of sleep, high stress, bad eating habits, and negative emotions.

When you take steps to release negative emotions, you raise your vibration. As a result, you feel better and you're naturally more optimistic—the perfect combination for believing. One of the simplest and most profound ways to raise your vibration is to release negative emotions as they arise throughout the course of your day.

Years ago, when I worked in the Internet industry, I used to suck on herbal stress-relief lozenges like they were going out of style. I was so stressed and full of nasty thoughts that I wore it on my face. I remember walking past a construction site and hearing one of the workers shout at me. Expecting a catcall, I immediately quickened my pace and my thoughts turned even nastier. However, I stopped in my tracks when I heard, "Smile, it can't be that bad." I looked the worker straight in the eye, and he seemed so earnest and well-intentioned that I couldn't help but return his smile.

Once I learned to quickly release negative emotions, my stress levels melted away faster than a lozenge on my tongue. The first thing I had to do was take responsibility for my emotions. If you want to let go of negative emotions, you can't blame your bad mood on circumstances, and you most certainly can't blame anyone else for your feelings. Only *you* have complete control over your feelings. No one else does. It is a responsibility, but it's also extremely empowering because it gives you a way to support the natural flow of qi in your body.

The Replace It Method

One of my favorite ways to clear out negative emotions and keep my qi flowing is to use what I call the *Replace It Method*. This simple process helps you release emotions as they come up so they don't get stuck in your body, muck up your qi, and drain your energy.

It's okay to have nasty feelings and express them. That's normal. It's human nature to experience a wide range of emotions, not just the happy ones. However, it is so much better for your health if you can release the negative ones as soon as possible. When you do, you also release the tension in your body that constricts the flow of qi.

Your body is quite resilient and can handle fluctuations in emotions—even extreme ones. Your body can handle *temporary* disruptions to the flow of qi. It just can't handle it when you bury the emotions deep inside or hold on to them for an extended period of time because then the qi constriction is never released. Let the negative emotions go, and your body can naturally return to balance because qi always wants to flow the right way.

The Replace It Method is super easy to practice because there are only two steps:

1. Become aware of the emotion.
2. Replace the emotion.

Step 1: Become Aware of the Emotion

Imagine you're driving along when suddenly a car cuts into your lane and you have to slam on the brakes. Nothing gets your adrenaline pumping faster than a perceived threat to your safety, especially if it's because someone else is being an inconsiderate jerk. You're fuming. What do you do?

1. First, you have to be aware of the emotion and have enough presence of mind and discipline to step outside yourself to approach the situation with a little bit of detachment. Pretend you're an impartial witness as opposed to the "victim," or maybe even the perpetrator!

2. Next, acknowledge the emotion. State the obvious, such as, "I am feeling angry."

3. Now comes your moment of empowerment because you assert that you have control over how you feel. Ask yourself, "Do I want to continue feeling this way?"

4. If you answer no, then move on to the next question. If you answer yes, ask yourself, "What is the benefit of staying in this emotion?" Sometimes there are benefits. For example, if you have a tendency to never express your anger, then it may be beneficial for you to wallow in it and curse like a famous chef on a reality TV cooking show.

   Even as you do this, maintain a sense of detachment where you are a witness to your actions, thoughts, and feelings. In this impartial state, start listing the reasons why it's good for you to stay mad. You'll probably notice your anger starts dissipating when you do this because it's hard to hold on to the negative when you're looking for the positive.

5. Once you decide that you no longer want to continue feeling the emotion, ask yourself, "How is this emotion affecting my body?" Do you feel pain or discomfort? A lump in your throat? A knot in your back? Pay attention to where you are feeling tension in your body because that's where you're constricting the flow of qi.

6. After you have finished taking inventory of the impact on your body, the final question to ask yourself is, "Do I want to keep doing this to my body, and is it really serving me?" Viewed from this perspective, your answer will most likely be a resounding *no!*

By being aware of your feelings and taking stock of how they affect your body, you are essentially short-circuiting the emotion. After you neutralize it, you can then switch gears by shifting to positive feelings that raise your vibration and get your qi flowing smoothly again.

Step 2: Replace the Emotion

Here's where the fun begins. You get to choose how you would rather feel instead. Replace those negative thoughts and emotions with a smorgasbord of good feelings that raise your vibration and boost your energy levels.

- **If you want to feel calm and clear . . .**

    Empty your mind and let all thoughts float away like clouds. Focus on your breathing. Take deep breaths to calm yourself down and divert your attention away from the negative situation.

- **If you want to feel focused and aligned . . .**

    Use a motivating goal. What do you want to achieve in life? Is there something that you desire and are working toward? Or is there something that you really want, such as a new home?

    When you focus on the goal, it helps you disperse any negative feelings that keep you from reaching your goal. In fact, any type of negativity is going to push away what you want in life because it lowers your vibration and drains your life force.

But when your life force is charged and your vibration is high, then you can attract the good things in life, things with a matching high vibration. So when something irks you, all you have to do is remember your goal and ask yourself, "Do I want this to stop me from getting what I want?" This will help you release negative emotions really fast.

- **If you want to feel love and joy . . .**

    Replace the negative feelings with a treasured memory. Remember a happy time spent with someone you love. You can use a happy memory to reactivate feelings of love and joy.

    You see people do this all the time at funerals. While the eulogy is read, there's so much pain and sadness. However, as soon as the speaker starts recounting a funny story or happy memory about the dearly departed, suddenly the energy in the room completely changes. People start laughing and smiling. The grief has been replaced with joy.

- **If you want to feel grounded and connected . . .**

    Tap into the energy of Mother Nature. Instead of feeling grumpy, sad, or fearful, place your hand on a tree trunk and feel its energy. You might not feel anything the first few times you try this, but with practice, you'll start to notice how your vibration feels chaotic and unbalanced compared to the stillness and rootedness of the tree's energy.

    Once you notice the difference, all you have to do is imagine your own energy matching the tree's energy. Basically, you're using the tree to recalibrate the frequency of your life force energy. It's like nature's tuning fork.

- **If you want to feel happy and uplifted . . .**

   Express gratitude and feel love and appreciation for everything in your life right now. No matter how crappy you're feeling, there is something for which you can express appreciation and gratitude—even if it's the smooth blink of an eyelid. Before you roll your smoothly blinking eyes at me over this example, consider that someone with eye tics would likely be extremely grateful if their twitching stopped.

   By taking a moment to appreciate how amazing your body is, you'll discover that there's a lot more going right than going wrong. So, what's working in your body? What's good about your life? I'm sure you'll easily come up with things to appreciate once you get started.

Keep It Up

You may have to cycle through the Replace It Method a few times to shake a strong emotion, but eventually it will start to fade away. If you find yourself getting sucked back into the negativity later, simply repeat the process.

As you practice regularly, it will become a habit. While you will still experience negative emotions, you'll let go of them much faster. Things that you might once have fumed over for weeks will be released in days. Something that could have wrecked your whole day will be gone in minutes.

I often tell people that the secret to my health and happiness isn't that I don't experience negative emotions like stress, anger, frustration, or sadness. It's that I let go of them very quickly. Now you can, too.

Belief into Action

As you continue practicing the Replace It Method, you'll notice over time that your energy feels lighter and your mood feels brighter. When you raise your energetic vibration, your qi will flow more smoothly, and you'll be more likely to take action to improve your health and well-being.

As you raise your vibration, you'll start seeing how your thoughts turn into tangible actions. For example, if one of your affirmations was "I have time to exercise," you'll get creative about finding more time. Maybe you'll cut down on random web surfing to free up ten minutes a day, or you'll get out of the car and do some stretches while waiting to pick up your kid from an after school activity.

When you raise your vibration, you also start appreciating yourself more, which leads to being kinder and more loving to yourself. This feeds on itself—the more you love and appreciate yourself, the more you love and appreciate yourself. You'll make choices that support your health and happiness. Plus, you'll follow through with action.

Now that you've learned the basic principles of the first catalyst to revolutionize your health—shifting the mind to heal the body—you understand a crucial foundation of healing: Health isn't a one-time decision. It is a continual choice made not just through your actions, but also by what you are thinking and feeling in each and every moment.

Your thoughts and emotions influence the flow of energy in your body. When you choose to dwell on negative thoughts, you're really choosing disharmonious qi because your feelings adversely affect the proper flow of qi. If a disharmony is not cleared at the energy level, then it can transform into disharmony at the physical level, which manifests as disease and discomfort.

The good news is that it's not that difficult to bring things back into balance. When you are choosing positive feelings, you are choosing ease, flow, and harmonious qi. So be vigilant when choosing your thoughts because that's how you choose health and vitality in every moment.

Congratulations! You're well versed in the first catalyst to healing and have the understanding and tools you need to shift your mind to heal your body. So let's continue on to the very powerful second catalyst—healing with energy—where we'll dive deeply into the secrets of Chinese foot reflexology.

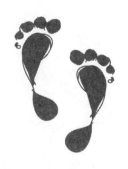

THE SECOND
CATALYST

HEALING WITH ENERGY

CHAPTER 6

HEALING WITH ENERGY

Now that you understand how to shift your mind to heal your body, are you ready to learn how to heal with energy? What's that? I can't hear you.

Imagine me onstage—a tiny Asian woman—stepping boldly across the platform. As I leap onto the podium, I pump my fists in the air and scream, *"Who wants to heal with energy? Let me hear ya!"* The crowd rises to its feet and roars.

Okay, please *un*-imagine that. There is a misperception in our society that having energy is about expending energy in order to show off how much you have. We think high-energy people are those who can work a crowd, or who bounce off the walls like a monkey in a room full of bananas.

I'm here to tell you that energy healing and living your life full of vibrancy is something entirely different. It's not a big display of action. It's actually something very personal and internal. Sure, you can have lots of energy, and you may love pumping your fists in the air—or not—but that's not how you cultivate your qi.

To the uninitiated, energy healing may seem like voodoo magic or witchcraft. When I was studying acupuncture, several of my classmates and professors told me they had met people who referred to Chinese Medicine as witchcraft. Aside from a deep love of a certain late-'90s television show featuring a teenage vampire slayer whose best friend was a witch, I can't say I know much about magic. And since that show was pure fiction, let's say my witchcraft knowledge is pretty much zero.

However, I *do* know about energy healing. To understand how to heal your body with energy, we first need to go over a few of the core principles of Traditional Chinese Medicine, and then I'll explain how they relate to Chinese reflexology.

Let's start by taking a little journey into Eastern philosophy, beginning with yin and yang. You've probably seen a yin yang symbol before, most likely emblazoned on a silver ring at a music festival during your college days. Admittedly, I was tempted to get the matching pendant, but when I was in my 20s, I really had no clue what a yin yang represented. Being Asian, I figured I should learn, so I bought a book on Taoism. It was my first introduction to Eastern philosophy, yet it felt like I had arrived home. Twenty years later, I still have that very book sitting on my bookshelf.

Yin and Yang and Your Body

In Chinese philosophy, yin and yang are a way to categorize everything in the world and the universe. A yin yang looks a bit like two fish swimming in a circle—one white and one black. The black fish is yin, and it represents female energy, darkness, earth, and cold. The white fish is yang, and it represents male energy, light, heaven, and heat. Inside each fish, there's a small circle of the opposite color.

This visual symbol embodies the relationship between yin and yang. There's a little yin in the yang, and a little yang in the yin. Where one ends, the other begins. They are constantly transforming from one into the other. This creates a state of dynamic balance, and thus yin cannot exist without yang, and vice versa.

In one of the many paradoxes in Chinese philosophy, even though something may be categorized as yin, it can also be categorized as yang. It all depends on what you're looking at in relation to something else because yin and yang have a relative relationship.

For example, Lady Gaga is yin when compared to a burly wrestler. However, if you were to compare her to someone more girly like Britney Spears, then Lady Gaga would be yang.

You could even categorize Lady Gaga's different looks and styles as yin or yang. Sometimes she's fully embracing her feminine side, and other times she is more masculine or yang when she's sporting an androgynous look. It's all relative, meaning that the same person or thing can be yin sometimes and yang at other times.

Yin and yang can also be used to describe your body. In Traditional Chinese Medicine, yin refers to the blood and fluids, whereas yang refers to qi and life force energy. Yin and yang need to be in balance in order for your body to be in balance. An excess or deficiency of either element will result in disharmony in the physical body.

Even though yin and yang are opposites, they are not mutually exclusive. Chinese philosophy views the two elements as mutually dependent. Thus, when you balance one of these elements, you help to bring the other back into balance. This is what makes energy healing so powerful. When you heal with qi, you're actually healing from both sides of the equation. Supporting the body's yang helps support the yin, which then helps the yang, and the cycle perpetuates.

Chinese Reflexology for Harmonizing Your Qi

The concept of qi is one of the cornerstones of healing in Traditional Chinese Medicine. Qi flows through your body just like blood circulates through your veins and arteries. Similar to how we have a circulatory system for blood, our bodies have a network of energy pathways for the flow of qi. The human body has 12 primary meridians or channels for qi to flow through. They are named by their associated organs:

1. Bladder

2. Gall Bladder

3. Heart

4. Kidney

5. Large Intestine

6. Liver

7. Lung

8. Pericardium

9. San Jiao or Triple Burner

10. Small Intestine

11. Spleen

12. Stomach

It's important to note that Traditional Chinese Medicine has a much broader perspective when referring to an organ. It includes the energy meridian, as well as the yin and yang elements of the organ. Because there's so much to say about each primary meridian, I'll share more of this ancient wisdom in the following chapters in the "According to Chinese Medicine" sections for the reflexology points associated with the energy meridians.

Special Note for Grammarians and Spelling Whizzes

You may have noticed that *Gall Bladder* appears to be spelled incorrectly because it is written as two words. This is actually the Chinese Medicine convention for referring to the Gall Bladder meridian. I find it a bit odd myself, but for consistency, I will use this spelling when I am talking about the Gall Bladder as it relates to TCM, and I'll use *gallbladder* when I am not referencing Chinese Medicine.

Another thing you may notice is that the organs for the primary meridians are capitalized throughout this book. Again, I am following TCM conventions. These organs will appear capitalized when I am referencing them in the context of Chinese Medicine. Otherwise, they'll appear in lowercase—unless, of course, they start a sentence!

The Flow of Qi in Your Body

When your qi is flowing as it should, your body is in a state of dynamic balance just like a yin yang. You feel energized, alive, and healthy. However, if the flow of qi is disrupted and not brought back into balance, this disruption will eventually manifest as *dis-ease* in your body.

For optimal health, you need a balanced amount of qi and blood flowing smoothly throughout your entire body, and that's where Chinese reflexology can help. Because your body's energy meridians pass through the feet, your feet house the master control points for harmonizing the flow of qi.

This makes the feet *a microcosm of the body as a whole.* If you put your feet together and imagine a human outline superimposed over the soles, you get an approximate location of your Chinese reflexology points.

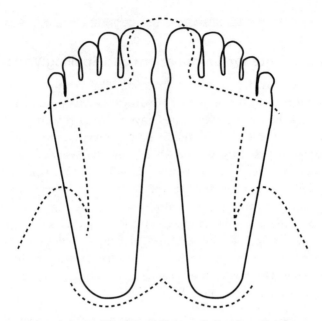

Approximate Location of Chinese Reflexology Points

Taking a look at the big toes in this diagram, you can see that this is where the reflexology points for the head and face are located. As you move down the sole of your foot, it's like taking a journey down your body, too. For example, right below your toes, on the ball of your foot, is the Lung point, and as you go farther down, you'll come across the organs for your digestive system. There are dozens of Chinese reflexology points on your feet, and each of these points corresponds to a different area of your body.·

How to Find Qi Disharmonies in Your Body

In order to diagnose qi disharmonies, a practitioner of Traditional Chinese Medicine will make a number of observations. They'll look at the color, size, shape, and coating of your tongue; feel for subtle differences in your pulse; and even take note of characteristics such as your body shape, your face color, and the sound of your voice.

They'll also ask a series of personal questions, including some that are rather embarrassing to answer. When I was an intern at the university clinic, I found some of the questions were also embarrassing to ask, especially the ones that got into describing the qualities of various bodily excretions.

After taking in all of this information, the practitioner will then identify which *zang fu* organ patterns match the person's signs and symptoms. Zang fu patterns are classifications for disharmonies in the body related to different energy meridians.

Phew, pretty complicated, huh?

Fortunately with Chinese reflexology, it's much easier to determine where there are energy disharmonies in your body. It's so simple that you can do it for yourself. All you have to do is feel your feet. If you find a reflexology point that feels sensitive or hard to the touch, this indicates an energy imbalance in the corresponding area of the body.

Energy blockages tend to feel like a hard buildup, almost like a callous *under* the skin. Disharmonies can also feel like small crystals in the feet. Sometimes they feel like grains of sand, and other times they feel like tiny pebbles. These crystals are a buildup of uric acid in the feet. The more crystals there are, the more likely that the qi disharmony has been going on for a very long time.

If a person is currently experiencing a physical ailment, the corresponding reflexology point will always feel sensitive. For example, someone with a shoulder injury will have a sore reflexology point for their shoulder. Past issues will also show up as sensitive reflexology points. After the shoulder has healed, if there's still scar tissue in the area, then the reflexology point will reflect this.

It's also possible to have a sensitive reflexology point without having any physical symptoms or issues. It takes time for a qi disharmony to show up in the body, so the energy disruption may only be at the early stages. This is an ideal time to practice Chinese reflexology because it's so much easier and quicker to restore balance when only the energy is affected.

Sensitive points can also indicate deep emotional pain held in the body. I had a client who had an extremely sensitive Heart reflexology point. Tony had no known heart issues and a clean bill of health for his heart from his doctor. However, when we delved into the emotional roots, we uncovered long-standing childhood pain held deeply within his heart. When the pain was released, his Heart reflexology point was no longer as sensitive.

Negative emotions such as pain, sadness, fear, anger, shame, and guilt disrupt the flow of qi. Release the emotion and the flow of qi will restore itself—especially when it gets a good nudge from Chinese reflexology.

The Heart of Traditional Chinese Reflexology

At the heart of this style of traditional Chinese reflexology is a reflexology stick. This is a small wooden rod that tapers into a rounded point at one end. The tapered end is used to press and massage the reflexology points on the feet. A reflexology stick allows for stronger and more targeted stimulation. It hurts, but it works. This follows the Chinese cultural adage of *no pain, no gain*.

My father had a bottle of "ancient Chinese secret" herbs, which bore a striking resemblance to severed digits marinating in a murky liquid. The things that looked like floating fingers were actually Chinese medicinal roots. My siblings and I affectionately referred to this concoction as *stinky stuff,* for the obvious reason that it reeked.

In the car accident, the side of my head struck the car window after it ricocheted off my sister's head. As a result, I had a huge bruise on the left side of my head. It was quite sensitive to the touch. When I returned home from the hospital, my father brought out the bottle of stinky stuff and vigorously rubbed it on my head for over half an hour.

He ignored my pleas to rub more gently, insisting that he had to press hard in order to break up the bruising. In Western culture, this might be considered a mild form of torture, but in the Confucian hierarchy of Chinese culture, this was fatherly care at its finest.

What could I say? Dad was helping me heal. It was just really painful, almost as much as the accident itself. In retrospect, I do have to say that the herbal concoction worked its magic, as my head never had any issues after the accident.

A Chinese reflexology stick follows a similar principle. When I press with a reflexology stick, it allows me to apply more pressure (no pain, no gain!) in a more focused manner. This enables me to get a better sense of the energy disharmonies revealed through the feet. Using the tip of the stick also lets me feel for the tiniest crystals under the skin and thus break them up faster.

If you try to use your fingers to find these crystals, it's like pressing your hand on a mattress to find a pea underneath. The stick lets you easily feel for tiny crystals, and as you massage them over time, you start to break them up, just like water wearing down rocks in a riverbed. As the crystals dissipate, the energy blocks in the body clear, too.

The harder and more focused the pressure, the more intense the stimulation of the reflexology points and energy meridians in the body. This results in faster healing of energy disharmonies. When the energy returns to balance, the physical body follows. I find that using a reflexology stick is at least ten times more powerful for balancing qi than simply massaging with your fingers or knuckles.

Because a reflexology stick is so powerful at shifting qi, I do *not* recommend that you go out and get your own. A chain saw can cut through a piece of wood much faster than a handsaw. However, it wouldn't be safe to start hacking away with a chain saw until you've learned how to use one properly.

Another reason why I don't recommend you buy a reflexology stick is because most of the ones I've seen for sale are made out of exotic hardwoods from endangered trees. To me, the idea of ancient forests being razed so that someone can buy a reflexology stick for a few dollars runs counter to the concept of balance and harmony.

If we desire harmony within, we must make choices that support balance and harmony in nature and the world at large. For this reason, I enrolled in a woodworking class to learn how to hand-craft my own reflexology sticks from sustainably harvested wood.

When people discover that I make my own sticks, they often ask whether I will sell them one. I tell them that the sticks are not for sale because I only give them to students who commit to learning the complete system of traditional Chinese reflexology. This is because the reflexology stick is such a powerful tool for moving qi. It's critical to learn how to practice correctly so that you don't negatively affect the flow of qi in your body. If you massage the wrong way, you could send your qi in the wrong direction, which would be counterproductive to healing.

It takes time and commitment to learn how to locate and massage all of the Chinese reflexology points—there are about 50 points in total. That's why I teach a comprehensive online Chinese Reflexology Sole Mastery Program. The program takes several months to complete with support and guidance from yours truly.

However, I also teach a gentle method of Chinese reflexology. That is what you are learning in this book, on my blog, and in my introductory online workshops. With the gentle method, you use your fingers, knuckles, and thumbs to massage your reflexology points. No matter how hard you press, you'll never be able to press as hard as you can with a reflexology stick. So, if you accidentally massage the wrong way, the effect is so mild that once you stop, your qi will go back to flowing as it was before the massage.

That said, it is still *extremely beneficial* to practice the gentle method using your fingers, thumbs, and knuckles to massage the reflexology points on your feet. When you are massaging the right way, you are creating incredible momentum for restoring balance in your body.

Going back to our flowing river analogy, it takes a long time to build a dam, but a lot less to tear it down. All you need to do is poke a hole in the dam, and the flow of water will continue working away on the hole until it becomes bigger and bigger, and eventually the obstruction breaks apart. Once the dam is cleared, the river rushes through as nature always intended.

I generally recommend that people start with the gentle method first. As Chinese reflexology becomes a part of your daily routine, you'll become more disciplined and more connected with your body, and then you'll be ready to learn how to use a Chinese reflexology stick.

Consistency Is the Key

You receive the most benefit from Chinese reflexology when you practice consistently over time. It's always better to start off slowly and gradually add to your practice as you get more in tune with your body—increasing the time and intensity of the massage over several weeks.

By massaging your reflexology points regularly, you stimulate your energy meridians, and this helps balance the flow of qi in the corresponding areas of your body. Better flowing qi promotes improved blood circulation, which brings more oxygen to the area and helps to clear away wastes and toxins from the body. This is one of the ways that healing at the energy level transforms into healing at the physical level.

To restore the proper flow of qi, you have to stop doing the things that muck up your qi (such as holding on to negative emotions or overthinking things), and start doing the things that get it flowing again (such as releasing negativity or practicing Chinese reflexology). When you massage your feet regularly, small shifts can add up to big changes over time.

Of course, you're probably curious how long it takes from when you start massaging your feet to when you notice a difference in your body. The answer is that it's different for everyone. It's not up to your mind to decide; it's up to your body.

Your body may also heal in ways different from what your mind expects. I had one client come see me for muscle atrophy in his hand, but before his hand showed significant improvement, his allergies went away. Everything is interconnected, so trust that when you see improvement in one area, it's a good sign that the rest of your body is getting better, too.

Tell your mind to go on vacation so that you can get out of your own way and let your body do what it knows best, which is heal itself. The moment you begin massaging your feet is the moment that healing starts happening at the energy level. The most important thing for you to focus on right now is creating a solid foundation for amazing health and vitality.

And that's how this book (and this section on healing with energy) is set up. You're walking through the steps to build your foundation, so it's important to follow the chapters sequentially and not skip ahead, even if it is really tempting to do so.

The reflexology points that you'll learn in this book are some of the most powerful healing points in this system. They're all-purpose points that are of the most benefit to the most people. But before we dive into these reflexology points, there are a few guidelines and precautions to pay attention to, and that's what the next chapter is all about. Read it!

CHAPTER 7

GUIDELINES FOR PRACTICING CHINESE REFLEXOLOGY

Chinese reflexology is very versatile—you can practice it almost anywhere and it's complementary with most healing modalities, including both alternative and Western medicine. That's because it helps strengthen and balance your qi, which supports the body's natural healing process. While massaging the feet is beneficial for most people, there are a few circumstances under which you should not practice reflexology, or you should proceed with caution. In addition, please note the following:

IMPORTANT

Chinese reflexology is not intended to replace medical care, nor should it be used as an alternative to medical advice from your doctor or health-care provider. If you have a health issue, please seek medical advice or treatment immediately. If you are not sure whether it is safe for you to practice reflexology, please check with your doctor.

When You Should __Not__ Practice Chinese Reflexology

Chinese reflexology is a holistic healing method with few, if any, side effects when you practice correctly and in moderation. This is especially true when you practice the gentle method of Chinese reflexology using your hands to massage your feet. That said, you should not practice reflexology, or you should proceed with caution, if any of the following apply:

- Pregnancy
- Heart condition
- Compromised immune system
- Diabetes
- Other chronic health condition, or prolonged use of medication

1. If you are **pregnant, do not** practice reflexology.

Because there are acupuncture points on the feet and around the ankles that stimulate labor, you should not practice reflexology on yourself if you are pregnant. Hey, it's only for nine months, so take it easy and look after yourself. After you give birth, then you can practice reflexology to help strengthen and rebuild your body. There's a belief in Traditional Chinese Medicine that the weeks after childbirth are critical for looking after your body. If you get lots of rest, eat well, and follow a TCM protocol, you have the opportunity to change your body's constitution and make it stronger.

2. If you have a **heart condition that requires you to check in with your doctor, do not** practice reflexology.

Chinese reflexology helps to move qi, which also increases blood circulation. If your heart is unstable, then the increased circulation may affect your heart. Thus, you should not practice reflexology if you have an acute heart condition (such as a recent heart attack), or if you have any heart condition where you need to check with your doctor before starting a new exercise routine.

If you're not sure, always consult with your physician first to see if it is okay for you to practice reflexology. It's a lot like getting the green light to exercise. If the doctor gives the okay, then use very gentle and light pressure, and massage the points for less than the recommended times. As long as it feels comfortable, gradually increase the massage time over a few weeks until you reach what is recommended.

3. If you have a **compromised immune system**, check with your doctor first. If you get the green light to practice, go slowly and gently.

If you are immunocompromised, be sure to consult with your doctor before practicing reflexology. After getting the clearance from your medical practitioner, you still need to proceed with caution. Chinese reflexology can help clear toxins from the body, but if your system is weak, you don't want to be clearing toxins at a rate faster than your body can handle—otherwise you may experience detox symptoms. These will be discussed later in this chapter.

4. If you have **diabetes**, practice gently and pay close attention to your feet.

For people with diabetes, use a very light pressure and massage the points for less than the recommended times. Diabetes can cause nerve damage that results in a loss of feeling in your feet. As a result, you may not realize if you are pressing too hard, and you could inadvertently give yourself a bruise or irritate the skin on your feet.

Diabetes can also weaken the kidneys. Because reflexology helps clear toxins from the body, if the kidneys are not functioning well enough to eliminate toxins through the urine, then one could experience detox symptoms, as discussed later in this chapter.

5. If you have a **chronic health condition, or have been taking medication for an extended period of time**, massage for less than the recommended times and use a lighter pressure.

If you've had a health condition for months or years (such as high blood pressure, chronic migraines, or allergies, to name just a few), or if you've been taking medication for an extended period of time, you may have a higher likelihood of experiencing detox systems—these are discussed later in this chapter.

Chinese reflexology helps to flush out toxins from the body, but in order to avoid detox symptoms, your body has to eliminate the toxins faster than they are released. If your body has been out of balance for a period of time, it may not be as efficient at eliminating toxins. Thus, it's important to start your reflexology practice gently as described in the "Best Practices for Chinese Reflexology" section in this chapter.

6. If you're **everybody else**, read this . . .

If you are an average person with no major health issues, it is very safe to practice Chinese reflexology. Basically, all you're doing is giving yourself a foot massage, and that's always a pleasant treat unless you have extremely ticklish feet. All joking aside, if you have any concerns, ask your doctor if it's okay for you to practice reflexology.

Possible Side Effects of Chinese Reflexology

Most people do not experience any side effects when massaging their feet, especially if they're only using their fingers, knuckles, or thumbs. The most common side effects I've seen tend to be minor and of short duration. They usually only occur when a person exceeds the recommended massage times, or if they are using a reflexology stick. Here are some of most common side effects and what to do if you experience any of them:

Sore or Achy Feet

If you have sensitive reflexology points, they may feel a bit achy for a few hours or days after an intense reflexology session.

This usually only happens when a reflexology stick is used, and if you have a large number of long-standing energy imbalances.

As long as you follow the recommended massage times in this book and use the gentle method, it is extremely unlikely that your feet will be sensitive afterward. You may notice tingly feet, but that's usually a pleasant sensation, and it's a sign that the qi is flowing through your feet.

In the event that you do notice any achy points on your feet, simply wait a few days until the soreness is gone, and then you can resume practicing reflexology. The next time you massage, use a lighter pressure and massage for a shorter duration.

Detox Symptoms

Improving the flow of qi can help clear toxins that have been held in your body for years. Practicing the gentle method of Chinese reflexology for the recommended times will help to clear toxins at a rate that your body can process. If your body's ability to eliminate toxins is weak, or if you have an abnormally large accumulation of toxins, then massaging your feet could possibly trigger the release of toxins faster than your body can handle.

This may result in detox symptoms such as headaches, fatigue, irritability, fever, diarrhea, rash, or other skin breakouts. That's why it is so important to get your excretory system functioning well so that you can clear toxins efficiently from your body. If you experience any of these symptoms, drink lots of water, eat light and healthy, rest and take it easy on yourself, and stop massaging your feet. Only resume practicing reflexology after the symptoms have passed, and massage more gently and for a shorter duration.

Detox symptoms usually only last a day or two. If your symptoms persist, you should consult with your doctor or health-care provider. Your symptoms may be caused by an unrelated condition (e.g., catching a cold) that coincidentally began when you started rubbing your feet.

Temporarily Protruding Veins

Reflexology helps stimulate the flow of qi, which helps improve the flow of blood in your body. The increased blood flow can cause your veins to be more visible, so that large blood vessels appear slightly raised or swollen, like they would if you were basking in the sun on a tropical beach. This effect is temporary, and your blood circulation will naturally return to normal so that the veins no longer appear swollen.

Skin Irritation

Skin irritation usually only occurs if a person massages a point beyond the recommended time or fails to apply a skin lubricant as directed. Some people are so eager to heal that they think the more they rub a point, the better it is for them. This is not the case, as too much rubbing can irritate the skin, especially for points on the tops and sides of your feet where the skin is more delicate than on the soles of your feet.

If you notice any skin irritation, stop rubbing your points immediately. Do not resume until the skin is fully healed. Apply a skin lubricant and always follow the recommended massage times.

Bruises on the Feet

Bruising can occur for the same reasons as skin irritation. If you notice a bruise, stop practicing reflexology and wait until the bruise heals before you resume. In the future, be more aware of your feet, and massage with less pressure and for less time.

Swelling in the Feet, Legs, Hands, or Arms

If you have a very sluggish or blocked lymphatic system, you may experience swelling in your feet or extremities. Stop massaging your feet and do some gentle exercises like stretching or light walking because the activity can help move lymph fluid through your body. Please see your doctor to get your lymphatic system checked out and to ask whether it is safe for you to practice reflexology.

Emotional Reactions

Because your mind, body, heart, and spirit are interconnected, massaging your feet can release buried emotions. What you think and feel can cause qi disharmonies, so when you clear energy blocks, you may also be clearing emotional blocks. If you do notice any strong feelings emerge after you massage your feet, be extra kind and nurturing to yourself. Take a break from the reflexology and begin again only when you feel emotionally ready.

Minor Short-Term Pain in the Corresponding Area of the Body

This is very rare, and if it does happen, it's usually only after you consistently massage your feet with a reflexology stick over several weeks. When there is an energy block in the body and you massage the corresponding reflexology point, the pain is a sign that the energy is trying to break through the blockage. This type of pain is mild and temporary, and dissipates on its own within a day or two. It's a bit like the stretching sensation you experience when you touch your toes but are out of practice. In this case, the energy is "stretching" through an area that was previously blocked. Wait until the pain passes before resuming your reflexology practice.

If the pain is intense, increases, or is long lasting, you probably have something going on that is unrelated to the reflexology. In this case, it is recommended that you get it checked out by your doctor right away.

Follow a Balanced Approach

If you notice any of the above signs or symptoms, stop practicing reflexology. Resume only after the symptoms have passed. I notice that people often want make up for years of poor health choices by rubbing the heck out of their feet. I appreciate their enthusiasm and desire to get better faster. However, it is possible to massage your reflexology points too much, which is counterproductive to healing.

Chinese reflexology is about restoring balance, so you should take a balanced approach to your practice. Change is subtle and occurs as you strengthen your body *over time* and *through consistent practice*. A little bit here and there is much more powerful than a single marathon session.

There is some flexibility for increasing the length of time that you massage a point, but before you do this, you should first be regularly massaging all the reflexology points that you'll learn in this book. Chapter 15, Putting It All Together, will give you direction on the best way to do this.

Best Practices for Chinese Reflexology

Okay, now that you know what not to do and what to watch out for, here's what you *should* do to get the best results from practicing Chinese reflexology:

1. **Start off gently.** When you are first learning how to massage your feet, start off gently. Use a light pressure and massage your feet for the minimum recommended time, unless you fall into one of the categories where you should proceed more cautiously. If that's the case, start out with half the recommended massage time and a very light pressure. If you're feeling fine the next day, then you can start increasing the massage time, always checking to see how you're feeling.

2. **Practice away from meals.** Massage your feet at least one hour before or after eating a meal. When your belly is full, your body's energy is focused on digestion, and the reflexology won't be as effective because your qi is otherwise occupied. When you practice away from meals, then your qi can flow to where it is most needed.

3. **Drink lots of water.** You can help your body flush out toxins by drinking lots of water before, during, and after your reflexology session. The water should be room temperature or, ideally, warm or hot, because this is considered optimal for the body in Traditional Chinese Medicine. Do not drink icy cold water as this is considered harmful to the digestive system, especially for the Spleen and Stomach. It can also cause abdominal cramps.

4. **Avoid alcohol.** Absolutely no alcoholic drinks! Alcohol affects the flow of qi in your body and is very hard for your body to metabolize. When healing your body, it is best to lighten your toxic load in order to assist your body in returning to balance. It's also good to eat lighter and healthier because you want to make things easier for your body so that your qi can be focused on healing.

5. **Always start with the excretory system.** Reflexology points in the excretory system (Kidneys, Bladder) should be massaged first to help your body excrete any toxins that may be released during your reflexology session.

A Note About Locating Your Points

Each person's body is unique, so the location of your reflexology points may differ slightly from what you'll read in this book.

But not by much—maybe by a smidgen here or there. If you want to be really precise, I'd estimate a variance of at most about an eighth of an inch, but then again, that also depends on the size of your foot!

There's a big difference between a size 5 woman's foot and a man's size 15, extra wide. That said, the instructions are intended as a guideline to help you locate your reflexology points. Don't worry about being perfect because that can really stress you out, which is the complete opposite of achieving balance. As you practice regularly, you will become more proficient at locating your points, and you will intuitively know exactly where the points are on your feet.

Ready, Set, and Go!

Okay, now that the basic guidelines are out of the way, *are you ready to heal with energy? Let me hear ya!*

Hee-hee, just kidding . . .

CHAPTER 8

CLEARING AND RECHARGING

KIDNEY, BLADDER, AND LYMPHATIC DRAINAGE POINTS

Moving qi through your energy meridians is like sending in the troops to clean your home—only instead of your house, it's your body that's getting a spring cleaning.

Better flowing qi improves the flow of blood, and this helps to clear away toxins and waste. And just like with any big cleanup, if you simply gather up the debris without having a process for hauling it away, then you're going to have an unsightly mess in front of your home.

That's why we always begin with the excretory system when practicing Chinese reflexology. It's one of your body's primary systems for clearing away toxins. You want your excretory system primed and functioning optimally in order to minimize the likelihood of experiencing detox symptoms such as fatigue, headaches, or irritability. Clearing out toxins efficiently will also help your body return to balance faster.

The Importance of Decluttering Your Body

Going back to our spring cleaning analogy, let's say that the garbage truck only came by once a month and it only collected one small bag per household. If you dumped several bags of trash at the curb every week, imagine the mountain of garbage that would accumulate outside of your home. You'd have heaps of trash bags with a thick cloud of flies buzzing overhead. The stench of rotting garbage would permeate the air and waft in through your open windows. This would result in some rather unsavory living conditions.

So, if the garbage truck only came by once a month, would it make sense not to bother with spring cleaning and simply live with the clutter in your home? You could move it around and hide it in closets, but eventually there would be so much waste that it would overtake your life. While the front of your home might look picture-perfect, the inside would be a mess. Garbage still smells, even if you can't see it.

You don't want the same thing happening in your body, where on the surface, everything looks fine, but inside your body is struggling. Thus, it's imperative that you clear out the waste.

After a spring cleaning, when your home is sparkling from top to bottom, doesn't it feel really good to live in it? When my family was selling our home, we were busy for weeks decluttering and scrubbing. The end result was a beautiful, open, and clear space that felt serene, peaceful, and extremely functional.

So, if garbage service only comes by once a month, you have two options. You either clean more slowly—meaning your house is messy for longer—or you get the garbage collectors to come by more often and carry away more trash with each visit. The key is to clear out the waste at a pace that matches the rate at which it is hauled away.

This also applies to your body. When there is a bottleneck for clearing out toxins, this can manifest as detox symptoms. A person might experience a bottleneck because their excretory system is not functioning optimally, or because they released a lot of toxins over a short period of time. If you've ever had a deep-tissue massage and felt achy and tired afterward, it may have been because the massage triggered the release of a lot of toxins all at once.

To minimize the likelihood of a bottleneck, you're going to give your excretory system a boost of qi so that it can work more efficiently. As you progress through this book with the gentle method of Chinese reflexology, you'll release toxins slowly over time so that your body doesn't get overwhelmed.

We'll cover two points from your excretory system—the Kidney and the Bladder. These two organs are critical components of your excretory system and they also have the added benefit of being primary energy meridians in Chinese Medicine. Massaging these points will help harmonize these meridians, and this has far-reaching benefits throughout your entire body.

Massaging your Kidney point also has the added benefit of boosting your life force qi. So, not only are you improving your garbage collection service, it's like you're getting a team of helpers to assist you in cleaning your home.

But wait, there's more!

Not only will you learn how to rev up your excretory system, I'll also show you a powerful reflexology point for your lymphatic system. As you learned in the You Are Here chapter, the lymphatic system plays an important role in filtering and removing cellular waste products and bacteria from the body.

The reflexology point for lymphatic drainage helps to improve the flow of qi through your lymphatic system, and this supports the flow of lymph fluid through your body. It's like opening up the double doors to your home so that the cleanup crew can easily haul the trash and clutter outside.

Chinese Reflexology Point for the Kidneys

The first point we'll begin with is the Chinese reflexology point for the Kidneys. You first learned about this point in Chapter 2, and now we'll cover it in much more detail. In Traditional

Chinese Medicine, the Kidneys and their corresponding energy meridian play an important role in health, vitality, and longevity.

What Your Kidneys Do

The kidneys are a pair of bean-shaped organs located in your lower back, on either side of your spine. They're a part of your excretory system, which also includes the bladder, ureter tubes connecting the kidneys to the bladder, and the urethra for passing urine out of the body.

One of the main functions of your kidneys is to filter your blood. The kidneys remove waste and excess water to produce urine. They also help regulate blood pressure and produce a hormone called erythropoietin, known as EPO.

If you've ever followed the sport of cycling and the Tour de France, you know that there was a big scandal over EPO and blood doping in the late '90s. This hormone stimulates the production of red blood cells, which theoretically enhances performance because more oxygen is being delivered to the body as a result. Share this trivia at your next social gathering, and you'll be the life of the party!

What Your Kidneys Do According to Traditional Chinese Medicine

As you learned in Chapter 6, the TCM view of organs includes not just the physical organ, but also the associated energy meridian and the yin and yang elements of the organ. For the Kidneys, this includes *Kidney yin* and *Kidney yang*, as well as Kidney jing.

Jing, also referred to as *Kidney essence*, is the substance from which all life flows, and it's stored in your kidneys. Think of it like a trust fund that has to last for your entire lifetime. If you spend it too quickly, your life ends sooner rather than later.

While it's perfectly natural for your jing to decline as you age, you do have control over how fast you use it up. Pushing yourself too hard, not getting enough rest, and eating a diet lacking in nutrients will result in a depletion of your jing. However, looking after your body and eating well can help conserve your jing.

There are two types of jing—*congenital jing* and *acquired jing*. You inherit congenital jing from your parents. When you are born, your parents make a deposit into your trust fund account based on how much energy they have to give.

If your parents are healthy and full of life, you'll get a bigger deposit than someone whose parents are sickly or lacking in vitality. It's just like money. If parents manage their finances wisely, then they have more to give to their kids. However, if the parents spend all of their money, then their children will receive a smaller trust fund.

Acquired jing is like the money that you earn throughout your lifetime. You receive it from what you eat and drink. If you eat healthy and nutritious food, then you've got extra money to spend for your day-to-day activities so that you don't have to draw down your trust fund as quickly.

You can also cultivate jing through practices such as tai chi and qigong, but there's another way that I believe is even more powerful—and that's connecting with the energy of the Universe. You'll learn more about how to do this when you get to the chapters on how to thrive by following your heart and soul.

For now, we'll start with your Kidney reflexology point because massaging this point helps to harmonize your Kidney channel, which is good not only for Kidney jing, but also Kidney yin and yang.

In addition to storing your jing, the Kidneys govern birth, growth, and reproduction, which is why infertility issues are usually rooted in weak Kidney function. The Kidneys also regulate water metabolism and produce marrow for your brain and spine. It is said that the Kidneys *control the bones, open into the ears, and manifest in the hair.* Thus, signs of aging such as osteoporosis, hearing loss, and gray hair are all associated with a decline in the Kidneys.

It is also said that the Kidneys are the *root of life*. I know when I first started studying Chinese Medicine, it seemed strange to me that the Kidneys were considered the root of life. Didn't they just filter blood and produce urine? What did that have to do with life force?

However, when I learned about EPO in anatomy class, it suddenly made perfect sense to me—and it totally blew my mind. The Kidneys really are the root of life. Let me walk you through this, because I bet your mind will geek out over this, too.

So, riddle me this—what is the one thing that you cannot live without? If you are deprived of this element, you'll die within minutes. Any idea? Nope, it's not food or water. And even though I talk about the importance of positive energy, the answer isn't love. And it's not money either!

If you guessed oxygen, you are correct. At the cellular level, oxygen is required for the process of respiration, which produces energy. Relating this back to the kidneys—this pair of organs produces EPO, which stimulates the production of red blood cells, and these cells transport oxygen throughout your body. So, this makes your Kidneys the root of life. Pretty cool, huh?

With all of these functions, and being the root of life too, you can see how the Kidneys are intrinsic to your health and well-being. Thus, the Kidney point is one of the most valuable reflexology points that you can learn.

How to Locate Your Kidney Point

IMPORTANT

The Chinese reflexology point for the Kidney is quite close to the acupuncture point *Kidney 1*. This point is sometimes used to induce labor in a pregnant woman who is past her due date. Do not massage this point or any reflexology points if you are pregnant.

When I first introduced you to the Kidney point, you learned a simplified method to get a general feel for where this point is located. Now you'll learn how to more accurately locate the point so that you can massage it to strengthen and harmonize your Kidneys.

The Kidney point is located on the soles of your feet. You have a Kidney point on each foot. The right foot is for your right Kidney, and the left foot is for your left Kidney. There is a series of steps to locate your Kidney point, so I'll break it down so that it's really easy to do. Simply follow these five steps to find your Kidney point.

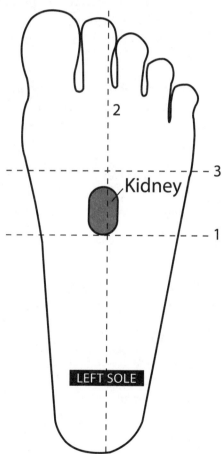

Chinese Reflexology Kidney Point

Step 1: Divide your foot in half horizontally

Imagine a horizontal line dividing your foot in half (Line 1). Measure from the tip of your big toe to the base of your heel and then divide this length in half.

Step 2: Divide your foot in half vertically

Imagine a vertical line dividing your foot in half vertically (Line 2).

Step 3: Locate the top inside quadrant

The two imaginary lines intersect to form four quadrants on your foot. The Kidney point is located primarily in the top inside quadrant. On your left foot, the Kidney point is located in the top left quadrant. On your right foot, the Kidney point is located in the top right quadrant.

Step 4: Imagine another line under the ball of your foot

The Kidney point is located below this line (Line 3) and above the horizontal divider (Line 1). Pull back your toes to help you locate the bottom of the ball of your foot.

Step 5: Place your thumb on your foot

Your Kidney point will be about as wide as your thumb. This is relative to each person, so your thumb is a good guideline for *your* Kidney point as opposed to someone else's. Place your thumb on the vertical halfway line, with about two-thirds of the thumb width in the top inside quadrant and the remaining one-third in the top outside quadrant. For example, if you're locating the Kidney point on your left foot, place most of your thumb in the top *left* quadrant.

And voilà, you've just found your Kidney point. Your final test to make sure you've found the Kidney point is to press into it with your thumb. Nine times out of ten, this is a supremely sensitive point for people. If it hurts, you've found it!

How to Massage Your Kidney Point

You can use your thumbs or knuckles to massage your Kidney point. If you're using your thumb, press the tip of your thumb pad into the point and massage in an up and down direction, where up is toward your toes and down is toward your heel. Work your way across and down the entire area for the Kidney. If you find a point that is especially sensitive, you can give it a little bit of extra stimulation by pressing deeper and rubbing your thumb in small circles on this spot.

To use your knuckle, take the index finger knuckle of your opposite hand and massage the point by sliding your knuckle up and down over the point. Because the skin on your knuckle is more sensitive than your thumb pad, it's a good idea to apply a bit of oil, moisturizer, or other lubricant to reduce friction so that the skin on your knuckle does not get irritated.

For a deeper massage, press in with your knuckle, lean in with your body weight, and hold for two to three seconds. Lift up your knuckle, move it along the point, and repeat until you've covered the entire point. After massaging your left foot, you can then massage the point on your right foot. Massage for 30 to 60 seconds per foot.

Chinese Reflexology Point for the Bladder

The Bladder point is a wonderful accompaniment for the Kidney point because it's the other major organ in your excretory system. In terms of spring cleaning your home, think of the bladder like a receptacle for refuse.

I know, that's not the most pleasant analogy for a part of your body, but sturdy trash bags and a good-sized bin are great assets in the cleanup process. A healthy bladder supports your excretory system.

For most people, the Bladder point is usually not as sensitive as the Kidney point. However, this point can be sensitive if a person has a history of urinary tract infections. While you may be thinking you're off the hook because you don't get bladder infections, think again because the Bladder point can be sensitive due to qi obstructions that *may not yet have manifested* in the physical body.

Many years ago, when I began my reflexology practice, I used to make house calls. One of my first home visits was for a woman who was a Reiki master. I arrived at Emily's home, and she had thoughtfully set up her own massage table to use during her reflexology session. The lavender massage table with energy crystals surrounding it was quite the contrast to Emily's cavernous industrial loft.

While massaging her feet, I noticed that Emily's Bladder point was unusually sensitive. She had no history of bladder infections, wasn't on any medications, was very health conscious, and lived a very natural lifestyle. So what was causing the problem?

As I glanced around her living space, I observed that her bed was located on a high loft with a ladder leading up to it. On a hunch, I asked her, "Do you ever have to pee in the morning, but you hold it in because it's really inconvenient to get to the bathroom?"

She exclaimed, "Yes, I do!" and nodded her head vigorously in agreement.

We had found the issue.

Ignoring her body's need to urinate disrupted the flow of qi in Emily's Bladder. She resolved to no longer lounge cozily in bed when she woke up, but to head straight for the bathroom first thing in the morning. By listening to her body and urinating when she needed to, she was helping to clear the energy block.

What Your Bladder Does

Generally speaking, when people refer to the bladder, they're usually referring to the urinary bladder, which is located in your lower abdominal cavity. This bladder is a sac that receives urine from the kidneys and stores it until you're ready to urinate. On the other hand, your gallbladder is part of your digestive system and it has a very different function. We'll cover it in more detail in an upcoming chapter.

What Your Bladder Does According to Traditional Chinese Medicine

The Chinese Medicine view on the Bladder is similar to the Western perspective in that the Bladder stores urine for excretion. However, the Chinese perspective sees the Bladder as having complex relationships with organs outside of the excretory system.

The Bladder receives fluids from the Small Intestine and requires qi and heat from the Kidneys to transform the fluids into urine. Because of this relationship, if there is a decline in Kidney function, which is common with aging, incontinence and frequent urination may occur.

In order to do its job, the Bladder also depends on harmonious qi flowing through the Heart, Lung, Liver, and San Jiao meridians. Who knew it required a symphony in order to take a proper piss in the toilet? Think about that the next time you go!

How to Locate Your Bladder Point

The Bladder point is a circle approximately as wide as your thumb. It is located on the inside edge and sole of your foot, just above the heel. About half of the point is on the edge of the foot and the other half is on the sole.

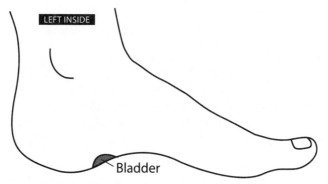

Chinese Reflexology Bladder Point on Inside of Foot

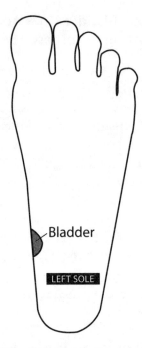

Bladder

LEFT SOLE

Chinese Reflexology Bladder Point on Sole of Foot

To locate the Bladder point, you'll first look for the middle of this point. Its center is located at the intersection formed by the curve of the top of the heel and the line where the skin and sole meet.

Let's start with your left foot. Use your thumb pad to feel for the top of the heel on the sole of the foot. After your thumb slides off the heel, follow the curve of the heel until you arrive at the inside edge of your foot.

Next, you'll identify the line that is formed when the skin and sole meet. Where the curve of the heel crosses this line is the center of the Bladder point. Place your thumb pad over the center and this gives you an idea of where your Bladder point is located.

While you only have one Bladder, you do have a Bladder point on each foot. Usually the sensitivity level for this point is the same for both feet, unless someone has had a pelvic injury or some other cause for asymmetry in their body.

How to Massage Your Bladder Point

To massage this point, sit cross-legged and rest your left foot comfortably in your lap. Press your right thumb pad into the point and massage in an up and down direction, where up is toward your toes and down is toward the base of the heel.

For a deeper massage, you can use the knuckle of your right index finger to press and massage the point, but be sure to apply a lubricant to the point to reduce friction on the skin of your knuckle. After massaging your left foot, go ahead and give this a try on your right foot and use your left hand to press into the point. Massage each foot for about 30 seconds.

Chinese Reflexology Point for Lymphatic Drainage

As you previously learned, the lymphatic system helps distribute white blood cells for fighting infection and also assists the body in filtering out wastes and toxins. It is similar to the circulatory system for blood in that it is composed of a network of vessels that move lymph fluid throughout the body. Not surprisingly, these two systems are also interconnected.

Capillaries are the tiniest blood vessels, and they have very thin walls. This allows for small amounts of plasma from the blood to exit the capillaries. Once the plasma exits the bloodstream, it's then referred to as *interstitial fluid*, a very lovely tongue twister. Go ahead and try saying that three times in a row really fast!

The interstitial fluid, interstitial fluid, interstitial fluid enters the lymphatic system through lymphatic capillaries, and then it's referred to as *lymph*. The lymph flows through the lymphatic system, where it is filtered in organs and lymph nodes. After completing its journey through the lymphatic system, lymph is returned to the bloodstream via the right and left subclavian veins, which are located near your collarbone. And then the cycle repeats.

The reflexology point for lymphatic drainage corresponds to the lymph nodes in the breasts and armpits, as well as the upper region of the chest where the filtered lymph returns to the circulatory system.

How to Locate Your Lymphatic Drainage Point

This one is super easy to locate, so we'll do a quick review of what you've already learned in Chapter 2. The lymphatic drainage point is located on the tops of both feet, in the webbing between the bones of your big toe and second toe. If you feel along the bones of these toes, you'll find that they form a V where they meet. The reflexology point begins at the base of the toes and continues to the point at the bottom of the V.

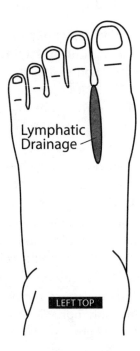

Chinese Reflexology Lymphatic Drainage Point

How to Massage Your Lymphatic Drainage Point

Because this point is on the top of your foot where the skin is more sensitive than the sole, apply some moisturizer or oil to reduce the friction on the skin when massaging. Use the knuckle of your index finger to press and stroke downward, away from your toes and toward the bottom of the V that's formed where the bones meet.

When you reach the bottom of the V, lift up your knuckle and place it back at the base of your toes and stroke downward again. It's very important to stroke in a *downward direction only,* as this is the way that the energy should flow through for this area of your body. Repeat for 15 to 20 downward strokes and then massage your other foot.

Points to Remember (bad pun intended!)

So now you know the importance of clearing toxins from your body through the powerful trio of the Kidney, Bladder, and lymphatic drainage points. They're the perfect triple-action combination to kick off your body's spring cleaning.

Here's a quick review of what we covered in this chapter.

1. Kidney Point

- **Benefits:** supports Kidney function, Kidney jing, and the excretory system for clearing toxins

- **Location:** on the soles of both feet, primarily in the upper inside quadrant, below the ball of the foot and above the horizontal halfway line, about the width of your thumb with about two-thirds in the inside quadrant and one-third in the outside

- **Massage Technique:** massage up and down (from toe to heel direction) with your thumb or knuckle, or press and hold with your knuckle for two to three seconds as you move across the point; apply lubricant if using knuckle to massage

- **Recommended Time:** 30 to 60 seconds per foot

2. Bladder Point

- **Benefits:** supports Bladder function and the excretory system for clearing toxins
- **Location:** thumb-width circle on both feet, half on the inside edge and half on the sole of the foot, at the intersection where the skin meets the sole and the top edge of the heel
- **Massage Technique:** massage up and down (from toe to heel direction) with your thumb or knuckle; apply lubricant if using knuckle to massage
- **Recommended Time:** 30 seconds per foot

3. Lymphatic Drainage Point

- **Benefits:** helps qi flow smoothly through lymph nodes in the breast and armpit areas and supports the lymphatic system for clearing toxins
- **Location:** on the tops of both feet, in the webbing between the first and second toes
- **Massage Technique:** apply lubricant and stroke with knuckle in *downward direction only* (away from toes)
- **Recommended Strokes:** 15 to 20 strokes per foot

CHAPTER 9

HARMONIZING THE HEART AND MIND

BRAIN, TEMPORAL AREA, AND HEART POINTS

Are you following your heart? Or is your mind in control of your destiny? It's pretty easy to figure out which is guiding you. All you have to do is to look at your life. If you're happy, healthy, and full of joy, and wake up every day full of energy, then your heart is leading you.

On the other hand, if you dread going into work or feel stuck in life, then it is probably your mind that's in charge. When the mind dominates your decisions, you make choices that are not in harmony with your heart and soul.

However, when things swing too far in the other direction, and the heart dominates decision-making, then people are ruled by their immediate emotions. They allow their initial feelings to drive their actions without tempering from the mind. This can lead to impulsive choices.

Ideally, your head and heart should work together. When the heart leads with support from the mind, then you achieve your highest potential. You are in alignment with your soul's calling, and your health and well-being soar.

Healing the Heart and Mind Connection
to Heal Your Body

I believe that the key to vitality is healing the relationship between the mind and heart. When we ignore our inner guidance, that's when our bodies create disease and discomfort—to draw our attention to what truly matters in life.

Most of my clients and students initially contact me because they want to heal their bodies. However, they often get more than they bargained for. When I work with people, not only does their health improve, but they also experience deep emotional healing and become open to following their passion. When the body, mind, heart, and spirit are aligned, the results are amazing.

Sara first came to see me because she had been suffering from anxiety attacks for more than five years. As she shared her story with me, she was often in tears as she was depressed and heartbroken over her grandmother's recent passing. The burden of grief was making her panic attacks worse. They had become unpredictable, striking in the middle of the night and occurring more frequently.

One of the first things I noticed while working on Sara's feet was how pale they were. After an intense Chinese reflexology session, most people's feet are warm and rosy due to the improvement in the flow of qi and blood.

However, Sara's feet remained cool to the touch, even after a 50-minute reflexology session. Based on her history of experiencing significant blood loss during childbirth, Sara was a classic case of what is known as *blood deficiency* in Chinese Medicine. While her immediate blood loss was addressed during childbirth, the TCM perspective is that an insufficiency of blood persists *after* childbirth. Thus, there was a physiological reason for Sara's anxiety and depression.

In Chinese Medicine, it is said that *the Heart houses the mind.* Because Sara had lost such a large volume of blood during childbirth—and it had not been addressed from a TCM perspective—she had an insufficient supply of blood to nourish her Heart. This led to mental and emotional issues because her weakened Heart was not strong enough to anchor her mind. When the mind is disturbed, its qi tends to float up and scatter. It needs the descending action of healthy Heart qi to counterbalance the upward rising of qi to the head.

For Sara, we addressed her qi imbalances and blood deficiency through Chinese reflexology and diet. However, I knew that to really turn things around, we needed to heal the connection between her heart and mind. Sara was a chronic worrier and overthinker. Her mind was affecting her Heart, and her Heart was not strong enough to balance her mind.

Her grandmother's passing had overloaded her system with stress. If we could reel in the worry and overthinking, we could give her Heart the space and time it needed to grow stronger; and this would naturally restore the balance between her heart, mind, and spirit.

I guided Sara into the Dragon Spirit space, where she was most connected to her inner guidance and the energy of the Universe. This enabled Sara to quiet her mind so that she could sense her grandmother's energy. Sara could feel that her grandmother was still there with her, albeit in a different form. This connection gave Sara peace of mind, which gave her Heart room to heal—thus restoring the balance between her Heart and mind.

Within a few months, Sara was a completely different person. Her anxiety attacks abated, and she was no longer overcome with grief over her grandmother's passing. Sara also changed her entire outlook and approach to life. She was able to let go of things that used to stress her out, and she became strong, grounded, and centered. When there was chaos, she was the calming presence. She became the rock of her family.

As her Heart grew stronger, Sara's connection with her inner guidance also grew, and she began listening to the whispers of her heart and soul. She started thinking about how she could pursue her passion for singing and creative expression. Sara hadn't even considered this as a possibility before, but now that it had entered her consciousness, she was considering what shape and form it might take in the future.

While Sara has only just begun her new journey, I know with all of my heart that she will achieve her goals, manifest her brilliance, and continue to experience more joy and vitality in her life.

You, too, can restore balance between your heart and mind. You, too, can hear your soul's calling and follow your passion in a way that works for you. You can fulfill your heart's desires and energize your life.

Your journey can begin with three remarkable Chinese reflexology points—the brain, temporal area, and Heart points—which we will cover in this chapter. This combination of points helps harmonize the flow of qi between your head and Heart.

As you continue your journey, be content with wherever you are in your progress. That's when the Universe will reveal your next steps, one at a time, to move you closer to your dreams. It is the mind that is focused on the destination, but it is your heart that draws you into the moment to appreciate where you are right now. And it is the two together that will take you to exactly where you want to go.

Chinese Reflexology Point for the Brain

The brain is in command of your thoughts, and what you *think* influences how you *feel*. This, in turn, shapes the choices you make, and the results of those choices are reflected in the life you create. Physiologically speaking, your brain is also in charge of all of the systems in your body.

However, we live in a society that emphasizes logic and left-brain thinking, so our minds start to get a little high on themselves, and this manifests as ego and arrogance. If you've ever thought that someone was an idiot, then your mind was being a little high and mighty.

Sometimes, it's good to take it down a notch. This doesn't mean that you denigrate your brain and all its wondrous talents. Instead, it's about restoring balance. Your mind has acted like an overzealous emperor, sucking up all the resources in the land. It's time to redistribute the qi because an overactive mind often results in a congestion of qi in your head. Yes, your body needs a leader, but it needs one that rules with compassion, benevolence, and for the greater good of the whole.

What Your Brain Does

So, what does your brain really do, aside from send a stream of nonstop chatter through your head? Well, the brain consists of four major sections: the cerebrum, cerebellum, diencephalon, and the brain stem. Each of these areas is responsible for different functions in your body.

The cerebrum is what we most often associate with thinking and consciousness. Different lobes are responsible for different functions, such as speech, memory, perception, and movement, to name just a few. The cerebellum helps you keep your balance and move your muscles. The diencephalon contains the thalamus, which is like a gateway for brain signals. And finally, the brain stem controls the autonomic nervous system—all of the processes that you don't consciously think about, such as breathing and the beating of your heart.

The brain is cushioned by cerebrospinal fluid and surrounded by a protective layer called the meninges. The outermost layer of protection is your skull. You can think of your head like a giant snow globe, where the outer shell keeps everything intact and the liquid helps protect what's inside from a sudden impact. (Hopefully, that's where the similarity to a snow globe ends, and your brain doesn't include a miniature replica of Las Vegas or some other tourist destination.)

How to Locate Your Brain Point

The brain reflexology point is located on the pad of your big toe. It encompasses the entire toe pad, much like your brain takes up most of the space in your skull. There are brain reflexology points on both of your feet.

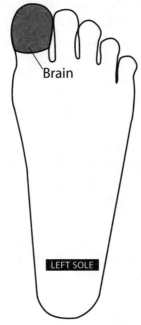

Chinese Reflexology Brain Point

Because your energy meridians cross over at the neck, the reflexology points on your feet are reversed for any part of the body from the neck up. Thus, the reflexology point for the right side of your brain is on your left toe, and the point for the left side of the brain is on the right toe.

How to Massage Your Brain Point

Use your thumb to press and rub your toe pad in an up and down direction, going up toward the tip of the toe and down toward the base of the toe pad. As you massage, move across the toe pad from one side to the other. Do this for 30 seconds and then repeat on your other toe.

I find that sensitive areas for the brain point tend to be concentrated at the base of the toe pad, which corresponds to the base of the skull. This makes a lot of sense given how much time people spending sitting at a desk, working at a computer, and hunching over their mobile devices. All of these activities can result in poor posture, which affects the smooth flow of qi to and from the head through the neck.

Often, the base of the toe pad, especially along the edges, will feel hard to the touch. If you were to press on this area with a reflexology stick, it would make a crunchy sound. I refer to these areas of long-standing qi obstructions as *crunchies*. A reflexology stick helps clear crunchies away faster, but you can also add extra massage time to help clear these energy blocks. If you feel a hard area on the base of your toe pad, add an extra 30 seconds of massage time for your brain point.

Chinese Reflexology Point for the Temporal Area

The reflexology point for the temporal area corresponds to your temples and the sides of your head above and around your ears. It also corresponds to your trigeminal nerve. Thus, this point is very beneficial for clearing stuck energy related to headaches and migraines.

If you're an overthinker or intellectual type, or if you use a computer a lot, this point will feel hard to the touch. If I were to press on your temporal area point with a reflexology stick, you would probably want to smack me because the point would be excruciatingly painful. Fortunately (for both of us), I don't happen to be anywhere near you with a reflexology stick right now.

What Your Temporal Area Does

The temporal area is significant because the trigeminal nerve is located here. This nerve has three branches, which send signals to and from your eyes, cheeks, and jaw.

How to Locate Your Temporal Area Point

The reflexology point for the temporal area is located on the inside edge of your big toe, between the big toe and your second toe. The point begins beside the toenail and extends all the way down to the base of your big toe pad.

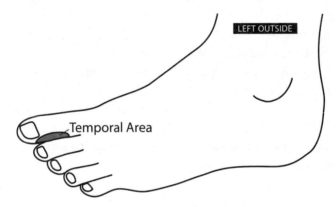

Chinese Reflexology Temporal Area Point

Similar to the brain point, your right toe is for the left side of your head and the left toe is for the right side of your head.

How to Massage Your Temporal Area Point

Use the thumb of your opposite hand to massage this point with a side-to-side motion, where your thumb moves from the top surface of your toe to the underside of the toe, and back again. Start beside your toenail and work your way down. I like to continue the massage right to the base of the toe as this encompasses a portion of the neck point, too. Very often tension in the temporal area is accompanied by tension in the neck.

When you get to the base of the toe, lift up your thumb, place it back at the top of the toe, and repeat. For this point, you always want to start from the top of the toe and work your way down to the base of the toe. This is important because the qi should flow downward from your head to your neck.

Because the skin on the side of the toe is more delicate than on the toe pad, apply a small amount of lubricant to reduce friction. Massage the point for 30 seconds to help smooth the flow of qi through the temporal area of your head.

I can always predict whether this point is going to be sensitive for a person based on their personality and occupation. People who are extremely analytical and work in jobs that require a lot of thinking tend to have extremely sensitive temporal area points. This is also true for people who are in their heads a lot or who worry too much.

I find that the sensitivity is usually most intense in the bottom half of the toe. It's an area where crunchies abound. While a reflexology stick is the tool of choice for slaying crunchies, you can also add additional massage time to help soften and dissipate these energy blocks.

If you're an overthinker (you *know* if you are), add an extra 30 seconds of massage time for this point, but do especially be sure to use a lubricant such as massage oil or moisturizer to reduce the friction. Also check to ensure that you are not irritating the skin on the edge of your toe.

And while a reflexology stick is ideal for dealing with crunchies, *consistent* massage is what matters the most. However, the real solution is to develop a regular practice of getting out of your head and getting connected with your body, heart, and soul. You're on this journey right now simply by applying what you've learned from this book to your life, so give yourself a pat on the back or do a high five in the air—or do both!

Chinese Reflexology Point for the Heart

The Heart point is an incredibly powerful reflexology point because it is a bridge between your physical body and emotional well-being. The heart is where people hold on to deep-seated emotional pain—the most profound and scathing moments in their lives, often going back to childhood. It's why our hearts feel vulnerable when we open up, because this is where our deepest pain is hidden. It's also where the greatest release can happen.

Tony came to see me for his arthritis, but I suspect his soul guided him to my reflexology practice for a more important reason—to help him release the pain in his heart that was holding him back from expressing his true brilliance.

When I first pressed Tony's Heart reflexology point, the sensitivity level was off the charts. Tony rated even the lightest touch on his Heart point as a 10 on a scale from 1 to 10. If I had pressed as hard as I normally do, this point probably would have rated as a 15. Usually, when a point is this sensitive, it means that there is a physical manifestation of disease or discomfort.

However, Tony had no heart issues. He had recently had a physical and his heart tests had come back clear. This led me to suspect that Tony held a great deal of emotional pain in his heart—so much that his Heart point was rating off the charts.

Tony worked in the corporate world, but in his heart, he really wanted to be an artist. He just had one significant problem—a creative block lasting for years. Tony was unable to draw freely from his imagination. Not since childhood had he sketched an image from his mind's eye. Growing up, he was constantly criticized and judged by his mother. As a result, he developed his own inner critic telling him that his drawings were no good.

In the Dragon Spirit space, we were able to journey back to Tony's childhood and rewire his internal programming. Being connected to his higher guidance enabled Tony to recall a memory of how he got into trouble for drinking all of the milk in the carton. Even though he was a growing boy and needed the nutrients, his mother scolded him harshly for finishing the milk.

This extended to all areas of his childhood where he felt barraged by judgment and constant criticism. It was this criticism that created the voice in his head telling him he was not good enough to draw. And it was the pain of a young child seeking approval, but receiving judgment, that he hid in his heart. This pain was held for decades deep within, and it kept Tony from following his heart, listening to his heart, and giving himself the freedom to draw freely.

Since finishing the milk epitomized the judgment and criticism he received as a child, I guided Tony through a process of retelling the event in his mind's eye. He saw himself gulping down the cold, white liquid without criticism, and it was the tastiest and most refreshing glass of milk ever.

I'm often thrilled at how quickly people respond to the energy healing of Chinese reflexology, but I'm always blown away by how fast they improve when the emotional roots of their qi disturbances are addressed. Such was the case for Tony. When I saw Tony the following week, the sensitivity level for his Heart point had dropped dramatically—going from a strong 10 to a rating of 6, a 40 percent improvement.

With reflexology alone (using a reflexology stick), this type of improvement usually happens over the course of several weeks. But for Tony, once he released the pain, it happened over the course of several days. Letting go of the past inspired a creative renaissance in Tony. He became a drawing machine!

After decades of being unable to sketch freely, Tony was doodling with abandon and spontaneity. On his subway ride to work, he brought a pad of paper and a marker. He would hold the marker loosely in his hand and allow the movement of the train to draw random lines on the paper. Tony would then use his imagination to transform these squiggles into fascinating sketches of landscapes, mythical creatures, and intriguing characters.

So that's what can happen when you uncover and release the pain held inside your heart. It gives you freedom to follow your heart. While your head may get caught up with how exactly to do this, your heart knows the way and it's guiding you right now. So let's discuss this amazing organ in more detail.

What Your Heart Does

Your heart is about the size of your fist, and it is located in the middle of your chest, off to the left side. Its main function is to pump blood through your blood vessels. The heart receives deoxygenated blood from your veins and then pumps it to the lungs, where it is oxygenated. The oxygen-rich blood then returns to the heart, where it is pumped into your arteries to deliver oxygen to the cells of your body. It's a continuous cycle, and your heart is at the center of it all.

What Your Heart Does According to Traditional Chinese Medicine

In Traditional Chinese Medicine, the Heart is not only an organ, but also a major energy meridian. It is said that the Heart governs the blood and controls the blood vessels. What this means is that the Heart helps circulate blood through the body, and it plays an important role in the health of the blood vessels. The Heart also takes the qi from food and transforms it into blood— yup, that's Chinese Medicine alchemy in action.

In Chinese Medicine, the Heart also houses the mind and spirit. If the Heart is weak and blood is deficient, this can lead to mental and emotional issues. On the other hand, a healthy Heart nourished with a rich supply of blood results in a healthy mind and spirit.

One of the most interesting things about the Chinese Medicine perspective on the Heart is that consciousness, intelligence, memory, and thinking are attributed to the Heart as well as the brain. The Heart and brain have a symbiotic relationship. It's just like the dynamic relationship between yin and yang, where the two counterbalance each other in order to function harmoniously.

How to Locate Your Heart Point

IMPORTANT

If you have an acute heart condition (such as a recent heart attack), do not massage your Heart point until your doctor confirms that it is safe for you to practice reflexology. If you have any heart condition where you need to check with a physician before starting a new exercise routine, then consult with your doctor first. When you get the green light to massage your feet, always use very gentle pressure and do not exceed the maximum recommended time.

The Chinese reflexology point for the Heart is an oval-shaped area located on the sole of your left foot. You'll find it in the top right quadrant below the ball of the foot and to the right of the Kidney point. Because the heart is located more on the left side of your chest, there isn't a Heart point on your right foot. To locate this point, follow the same steps you would for locating your Kidney point.

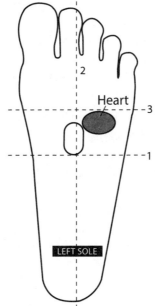

Chinese Reflexology Heart Point

Step 1: Divide your foot in half horizontally

Imagine a horizontal line dividing your left foot in half (Line 1). Remember to measure from the tip of your big toe to the base of your heel and use this distance to place the imaginary halfway line.

Step 2: Divide your foot in half vertically

Next, imagine another line dividing your foot in half vertically (Line 2).

Step 3: Locate the top outer quadrant

These two lines form four quadrants on your foot, and the Heart point is located in the top right quadrant of your left foot.

Step 4: Imagine another horizontal line under the ball of your foot

The Heart point is located below the ball of the foot (Line 3), to the right of your Kidney point.

Step 5: Place your thumb on your foot

Place one thumb centered over the vertical dividing line (Line 2) and just below the horizontal line under the ball of your foot (Line 3). Next place your other thumb to the right of the first thumb.

This gives a good approximation of your Heart point. It is wider than your thumb and its height is about half of the height of the space between the ball of your foot (Line 3) and the horizontal dividing line (Line 1).

However, your actual Heart point may be slightly wider, thinner, shorter, or longer because each person's body is different. If you have a wide foot, your Heart point may be wider. If you have a long and narrow foot, your Heart point may be longer and skinnier.

As you practice consistently over time, you'll get a better feel for where your Heart point is located. In the meantime, think of it like a coloring book where it is okay for you to color outside of the lines for this point.

How to Massage Your Heart Point

Use your thumb pad to massage this point for 20 seconds in an up and down direction, where up is toward your toes and down is toward your heel. Since it's okay to color outside of the lines, feel free to massage a little wider on both sides, going toward the Kidney point and all the way to almost the edge of the foot.

If you massage outside of your Heart point, you'll be giving your Kidney and Spleen points a few extra seconds of massage. That's okay for these two points. And you're going to learn in the next chapter the significance of the Spleen and the benefits of massaging this reflexology area.

Points to Remember

Balancing your heart and mind helps you reconnect with your body and be more in tune with its needs. The brain, temporal area, and Heart points are a powerful combination for promoting harmony between your body, mind, heart, and spirit. Here's a quick summary of the points from this chapter.

1. Brain Point

- **Benefits:** supports brain function, helps balance the Heart and mind, and clears energy blocks in the head
- **Location:** on the big toe pad of both feet
- **Massage Technique:** massage up and down (from tip of toe to base of toe pad) with thumb
- **Recommended Time:** 30 seconds per foot, extra 30 seconds for overthinkers

2. Temporal Area Point

- **Benefits:** helps to clear blocked energy in the temporal region and sides of head, pain relief for headaches and migraines

- **Location:** on the inside edge of the big toe for both feet

- **Massage Technique:** apply lubricant and massage side to side (surface to underside direction) with thumb from tip of toe to base of toe, reposition thumb at toe tip and repeat

- **Recommended Time:** 30 seconds per foot, extra 30 seconds for overthinkers

3. Heart Point

- **Benefits:** supports Heart function and balances the Heart and mind

- **Location:** oval-shaped area on the sole of the left foot, in top right quadrant below the ball of the foot and beside the Kidney point

- **Massage Technique:** massage up and down (from toe to heel direction) with thumb

- **Recommended Time:** 20 seconds

CHAPTER 10

Nourishing Your Body

Solar Plexus, Spleen, and Stomach Points

Imagine you own a really fancy car, like a Ferrari or Maserati. Would you cheap out on gas and use low-quality parts to maintain your vehicle? Of course not. So why would you do the same for your body? You wouldn't, right?

If you think of your body as a car, your excretory system is what cleans buildup in the engine, and your digestive system is what powers your vehicle. You want to optimize your digestion because that's what puts premium gas in your tank. It's what makes you go *vroom*!

Digestion: An Important Building Block for Health

Healthy digestion is the key to a healthy body. Many illnesses and chronic conditions can be linked to a disturbance in the digestive system. Sometimes the connection may not be obvious at first glance. This certainly was the case for Jordan.

He first came to see me about weakness and atrophy in his left hand. He also experienced tingling and numbness in both of his arms. Looking at him, you'd never know he had any health issues. He was big and muscular with tattoos on his arms. He looked like a tough guy until you got to know him and discovered he had a soft spot for his wife and kids.

The atrophy in his hand had persisted for years. Jordan couldn't make a tight fist; and when he held up his hand with fingers outstretched, I couldn't help but notice a slight tremor in his fingertips.

Over the years, Jordan had been bounced from doctor to doctor, as often as a ping-pong ball in a champion match of table tennis. He'd seen numerous specialists, and while they were able to conclusively rule out what *wasn't* causing the problem, none of them could tell him what *was* causing the problem, let alone how to fix it. The medical experts either referred him to yet another specialist or told him that they would monitor his condition.

Many years passed with no improvement. Jordan's fingers were beginning to curl into a claw hand, a common occurrence when the muscles in the hand waste away over a long period of time. While he'd been given many hypotheses for the cause of his symptoms, no one really knew the answer. But then again, no one had ever asked his feet. Sure enough, when I started massaging Jordan's reflexology points, a clear picture emerged.

All of the points related to the digestion of food were extremely sensitive. Taking into account Jordan's age, these points were much more sensitive than I would have expected. His feet indicated that a long-standing energy imbalance had manifested at the physical level in his digestive system.

In Chinese Medicine theory, it is said that the *Spleen governs the four limbs.* You'll learn more about the Spleen a little later in this chapter, but what this saying essentially means is that if a person's digestion is weak, then their limbs are not getting enough nourishment. This can result in weakness and wasting in the arms and legs.

Working with Jordan over the course of several months, healing occurred at the energy level through Chinese reflexology and shifting his belief structures. Jordan had spent so many years going from doctor to doctor that he had inadvertently given away his own power to heal himself by looking to others for healing.

As he shifted his beliefs, Jordan reclaimed his power to heal his body. He became proactive about making nourishing health decisions and chose to think thoughts that would support his healing. Jordan took ownership of his health, massaged his reflexology points daily, and slowly, but surely, he started to see improvement.

After years of witnessing a steady decline in the function of his hand, Jordan reached a turning point. His grip improved and the numbness in his hands and forearms went away. His wife remarked that she could see his fingers starting to lengthen and straighten. The claw hand was no longer a part of his identity.

Another change that occurred was that Jordan's allergies completely disappeared. He used to sneeze violently when he was exposed to traces of dog hair—even if the dog was nowhere nearby. But after a few months of massaging his feet regularly with a reflexology stick, Jordan no longer had an allergic reaction and his seasonal allergies went away, too.

His remarkable recovery highlights how important the digestive system is for your overall health and vitality. Poor digestion can be the root of many conditions, even those that may seem completely unrelated at first. When you improve your digestion, you give your body *the building blocks* it needs to heal. It's like sourcing the right parts to repair your Ferrari. You can give your body an energy boost to replenish your Kidney jing, but you can also give your body a physical boost by strengthening your digestion.

In Chinese reflexology, almost half of the points in this system are related to the digestive system. Let's get you started with three essential reflexology points for healthy digestion—the solar plexus, Spleen, and Stomach.

Chinese Reflexology Point for the Solar Plexus

Your imaginary Ferrari comes with a sophisticated electronic system for monitoring and managing your car's performance. In your body, the solar plexus takes on this role. It is considered to be the abdominal "brain" in charge of digestion. When you massage the solar plexus point, it's like turning the key in the ignition to activate the electronics in your car—only in the case of digestion, you're ensuring that the nerve center for digestive signals is up and running.

The solar plexus also has metaphysical significance. It is the location of your solar plexus chakra, a formidable energy center according to Hindu traditions. This chakra is associated with personal power, confidence, and a sense of self.

What Your Solar Plexus Does

The solar plexus is located just below the breastbone along the center line of your body. It is a dense network of nerves transmitting signals between your brain and numerous organs. It's like the Grand Central station for your abdominal cavity. Nerves radiate from the solar plexus to vital organs such as your stomach, spleen, and pancreas, to name just a few.

How to Locate Your Solar Plexus Point

This reflexology point is a small circle located on the sole of your foot. Even though you only have one solar plexus, there are two reflexology points for it—one on your left foot and one on the right.

To locate this point, first imagine a vertical line dividing your foot in half. Place your thumb on this imaginary vertical line close to the top of your sole. Then slide your thumb down the line until you feel a slight indentation just below the ball of your foot. This is similar to your chest, where your solar plexus is located in the depression just below your breastbone. On your foot, the depression may be slightly off center.

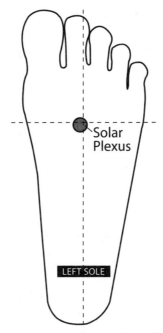

Chinese Reflexology Solar Plexus Point

How to Massage Your Solar Plexus Point

Press deeply into your solar plexus point with your thumb, and massage in small circles. Massage for a total of 15 seconds per foot. Alternatively, you can use the knuckle of your index finger to press and twist into the point. Turn your wrist back and forth as if you were jiggling a key in a finicky door lock, only you're unlocking the door to your personal power and true self. Hmm, something to ponder . . .

Chinese Reflexology Point for the Spleen

If the solar plexus is the onboard computer for your car's electronic system, then the Spleen is the engine. Just as the engine is the "muscle" in a car, the Spleen plays a critical role in strengthening your body's muscles. So rev up your engine by learning more about the Spleen.

Perhaps the best example I can give you of the importance of the Spleen is my own story. I used to be the epitome of *Spleen qi deficiency*. I exhibited all of the classic symptoms of having a low level of qi in my Spleen channel. These included a pale complexion, poor appetite, and scalloped edges on my tongue.

The other common symptom was feeling tired all the time. When I worked in high tech, I'd get home from the office and immediately fall asleep on the couch. I thought it was because of the long hours and stressful projects, but it was really due to Spleen qi deficiency.

I had also cornered the market on activities that were bad for the Spleen. These included overthinking, worrying too much, eating at odd hours, grabbing meals on the go, and snacking on cold food straight from the refrigerator.

Not eating enough protein also weakens the Spleen. For close to a decade, I followed a mostly vegan diet. I'm not here to pass judgment on what people should or shouldn't eat. I believe that it really depends on a person's constitution and personal beliefs. There is no one-size-fits-all diet.

For me, however, I needed more protein, and it felt like my body was craving animal protein. During the early weeks of my pregnancy, I was tired all the time. I'd spend the afternoon napping and then feel guilty about not being productive. I felt like I wasn't doing anything. My husband kindly and wisely pointed out that I was doing the most important thing ever. He said, "You're growing a baby."

After hearing his words, I embraced my lack of productivity. I spent a lot of time sleeping, eating, and reading a ton of baby books. I had a stack of pregnancy books that was almost two feet high. In one of the books, it listed a recommendation for the number of grams of protein that a pregnant woman should consume each day. I mentally tallied what I ate on a typical day and discovered that what I was eating had a lot less protein in it than I thought—I was getting about a third of the daily recommendation.

Later that day, I came across an article about how meat consumption was on the rise in China as its citizens became more affluent. The article mentioned the annual protein consumption per person *before* the rise in affluence. It was an eye-opener for me as I was consuming less than half of the "before" diet. No wonder I felt tired all the time.

I started eating more animal protein, and within days, I could feel a difference in my body. I felt like I had been craving meat for years, and now that my body was getting enough, it was soaking up the protein like a parched plant finally being watered. My energy levels soared, and I felt stronger and healthier than I had in years.

Being pregnant was a wonderful gift because not only did I appreciate the importance of eating enough protein, but the hormones made my brain fuzzy. It gave me *pregnancy brain*. I had it in spades, but the *momnesia* (mommy-induced amnesia, aka forgetfulness) served me well because it made me stop multitasking and worrying about things I couldn't control. I learned how to embrace living in the moment. Combined with eating at regular intervals, I'd say my pregnancy was the best thing for rebuilding my Spleen qi.

If you want to boost your Spleen qi, getting pregnant isn't the only way to do so. You can also massage your Chinese reflexology point for the Spleen. But before we delve into how to do this, let's explore what this amazing organ does for your body.

What Your Spleen Does

The spleen is located in the upper left side of your abdomen, close to your ribs and next to your stomach. It's part of the lymphatic system and plays an important role in supporting your immune system. The spleen produces white blood cells, stores blood cells, and also acts as a blood filter to remove worn-out red blood cells.

What Your Spleen Does According to Traditional Chinese Medicine

The Spleen is one of the most important organs and energy meridians for healthy digestion. The Spleen meridian is paired with the Stomach meridian, and they work together to extract qi from your food.

This particular qi is referred to as *gu qi*. This phrase is pronounced like a famous Italian handbag, only you add extra emphasis to the first syllable, drawing it out a little longer. Gu qi is the foundation for producing blood and other types of qi in your body. It also contributes to your acquired jing. Thus, it's like the money you earn for day-to-day spending so that you can preserve your Kidney jing. After transforming food into gu qi, the Spleen then helps to distribute it throughout the body.

The Spleen also transforms and transports fluids in the body. During digestion, the Spleen sorts out "clear" fluids for the body to use and then gets rid of the "turbid" fluids through the intestines. This helps keep mucous and phlegm at bay.

These are some of the most important things that the Spleen does in your body, but there are many more functions too numerous to mention. Literally, I could write an entire chapter about the Spleen, and in fact, many TCM textbooks contain one or more chapters explaining the Spleen and its functions.

What matters most for healthy digestion is to strengthen your Spleen qi. In addition, it is good to avoid doing activities that hurt the Spleen. Generally speaking, if you want to support your Spleen, eat balanced meals at regular intervals in a relaxed manner, don't overeat, and avoid consuming cold foods and drink as it's said that the *Spleen likes warmth and dislikes cold.* And of course, massage the Chinese reflexology point for your Spleen!

How to Locate Your Spleen Point

You'll find your Spleen point on the sole of your left foot. Locating this point is very similar to finding your Kidney and Heart points. First imagine a horizontal line dividing your foot in half between the tip of your big toe and the base of your heel. Next, imagine a vertical line bisecting your foot in half.

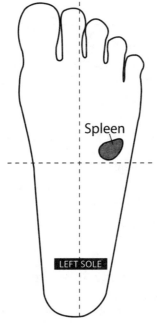

Chinese Reflexology Spleen Point

The Spleen point is located in the top right quadrant of your left foot. While most reflexology points can be eloquently described as round, square, or rectangular, the Spleen point is best described as a blob. To find your Spleen point, use your thumb to press deeply on your sole above the horizontal halfway line. Feel for the area that is most sensitive and that is your Spleen point.

How to Massage Your Spleen Point

Use your thumb to rub the Spleen point in an up and down motion, where up is toward your toes and down is toward your heel. If any area feels particularly tender, press deeply into the sensitive spot and massage in small circles. You can also use your knuckle to press and massage the Spleen point as long as you use a lubricant to prevent friction from irritating the skin of your knuckle.

If you're not 100 percent sure where your Spleen point is located, feel free to massage slightly wider than your best guess as long as you stay within the quadrant. Massage this point for 30 to 60 seconds.

Chinese Reflexology Point for the Stomach

By now, you know that the solar plexus is the onboard computer and the Spleen is the engine for your sports car. So, what's the Stomach? It's similar to the gas tank, receiving the fuel for your body, and injecting additives to enhance performance.

What Your Stomach Does

The stomach is a J-shaped organ located in the upper-left side of your abdomen. It receives the food that you've chewed up in your mouth. Did you know that after you chew your food into a gooey ball, it's then called *bolus*? One day, when you're playing a trivia game and this question comes up, you'll know the answer (you can thank me later). Bolus then becomes *chyme* in your stomach, where it is mixed with stomach acid and digestive enzymes. The chyme then passes to the small intestine for further digestion.

What Your Stomach Does According to Traditional Chinese Medicine

The Stomach is one of the 12 primary meridians in your body and it is responsible for what Chinese Medicine describes as the *rotting and ripening of food*. Basically, it breaks down the food you eat into nutrients that your body can use. The Stomach is also considered the *origin of fluids*. It derives fluids from what you eat and drink to be used by your body.

In addition to digesting food, the Stomach also has the responsibility of keeping the partially digested food down so that you don't upchuck it. If a person experiences excessive burping or vomiting, it is said that they have *rebellious Stomach qi* because the qi is rising upward and going in the opposite direction from how it is supposed to flow. Stomach qi is supposed to descend in order to direct food to the small intestine.

How to Locate Your Stomach Point

The Stomach reflexology point is located on the soles of both feet. You'll find it below the ball of your foot and toward the inside edge on both feet, right next to the Kidney point.

Examining your hand can help you locate this point on your foot. Take a look at the palm of either hand and touch your thumb to the tip of your pinky finger. Notice how there's this big fleshy area on your palm that moves along with your thumb. It's called the *thenar* of the thumb.

If you look at the sole of your left foot and flex your toes all the way back, you'll notice that your big toe has a similar fleshy area underneath. This is the ball of your foot, but it extends just a little bit farther down on the side where your big toe is, as compared to under your pinky toe.

Place your left thumb below your big toe "thenar" (it's technically not called that, but I think it's a good way to describe it) so that your thumb runs parallel to the ball of your foot, but with a slight upward angle. Line up the knuckle of your thumb with the inside edge of your foot. The area that your thumb is covering is a good approximation of the location of the reflexology point for your Stomach.

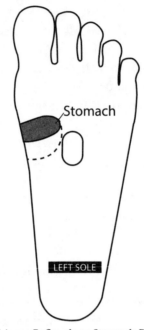

Chinese Reflexology Stomach Point

The Stomach point is actually larger than the first segment of your thumb (see dotted outline in the diagram). However, because this point overlaps with a couple of other digestive points, it's best to focus on just the top portion of the Stomach. This will minimize the chances of experiencing detox symptoms because the other two digestive points (pancreas and duodenum) are often extremely sensitive for many people.

How to Massage Your Stomach Point

Since your thumb is already in the right place, simply pivot your thumb 90 degrees, and use your thumb pad to massage your Stomach point in an up and down direction, where up is toward the toes and down is toward the heel. Massage for 15 seconds per foot.

Don't be surprised if you hear a grumbling sound in your stomach when you massage this point. Your stomach is responding to the increase of qi and blood flowing through the area. I often hear a gurgle when I rub my own digestive points.

Points to Remember

Hooray! You now know three amazing reflexology points—the solar plexus, Spleen, and Stomach—to rev the engine of the priceless Ferrari that is your body. Here's a summary of these powerful fuel-injection points for turbocharging your digestion.

1. Solar Plexus Point

- **Benefits:** supports abdominal brain (nerves running through solar plexus to organs in the abdominal cavity)
- **Location:** small circle on the soles of both feet, on or near the vertical center line, below the ball of the foot
- **Massage Technique:** massage in small circles with thumb, or press and twist with knuckle
- **Recommended Time:** 15 seconds per foot

2. Spleen Point

- **Benefits:** supports Spleen function for digestion and distribution of nutrients
- **Location:** "blob" on the sole of the left foot in the top right quadrant above the horizontal halfway line
- **Massage Technique:** massage up and down (toe to heel direction) with thumb or knuckle; apply lubricant if using knuckle to massage
- **Recommended Time:** 30 to 60 seconds

3. Stomach Point

- **Benefits:** supports stomach function for digesting food and ensuring that qi descends to direct food toward small intestine
- **Location:** circular area on the soles of both feet below the ball of the foot on the inside edge of the foot, beside Kidney point
- **Massage Technique:** massage top portion up and down (toe to heel direction) with thumb
- **Recommended Time:** 15 seconds per foot

CHAPTER 11

RESTORING BALANCE

LIVER, ADRENAL GLAND, AND PITUITARY GLAND POINTS

Stress is insidious and sneaky. We believe we can handle it, so we don't acknowledge the tension until our bodies start to break down. Stress denial can happen to anyone. Just because you drink green shakes and go to yoga class does not mean you're in the clear. In fact, some of the most high-strung people I've ever met did both of these things. While diet and exercise are important components of self-care, it is equally important to pay attention to your body and take care of it before problems arise.

That's why your reflexology points are so awesome. They will let you know right away when there's an issue—even if you think you've got everything under control and that you can handle the stress.

Long before you see physical symptoms, such as weight gain, exhaustion, heart palpitations, insomnia, or high blood pressure, your feet will let you know that the stress is too much to handle. So even though you may pat yourself on the back for going to the spa, your feet will tell you that a single mud wrap isn't going to make up for weeks of overtime. With feedback from your feet, you gain insight into what your body is able to handle and what it needs you to do (or stop doing) in order to thrive.

In this chapter, you'll learn about the Liver and adrenal gland points. These points give you a heads-up when your stress levels are getting out of hand—and into your feet. You'll also learn about the pituitary gland point, which is very beneficial for your endocrine system. Combined, these three reflexology points are a powerful trio for releasing the effects of stress and bringing your body back into balance.

The Importance of Releasing Stress Today, Not Tomorrow

Nothing disrupts your sense of balance faster than stress and worry. If you're stressed, your qi's messed. Instead of heading toward burnout, it's better to turn things around at the energy level *before* your health suffers.

However, often when you're in the thick of things, you ignore the early warning signs and, as a result, you think that you can put off self-care until later. I know because I did this myself. When I worked in the Internet industry, I was burning the candle at both ends for many years. I only made changes when my health suffered. It was rather ironic because I had always considered myself to be a Type B personality with a laid-back attitude toward life.

Logically speaking, you would wonder why someone would not value their health more, but it happened to me, and I see it happening all the time with other people, too. I once taught a Chinese reflexology workshop at the headquarters of a very well-known high-tech company. I was invited to speak at an employee-organized special interest group within the company. The group's focus was on personal growth, spirituality, and holistic health. You would think if anyone should have been stress-free and into self-care, it would have been this group of people, but that's not what I saw.

When I arrived at the campus (that's what the cool kids call their offices in Silicon Valley), I experienced an eerie sense of déjà vu. It reminded me of when I worked in high tech, except instead of heading to my cubicle with a laptop, I was heading to a presentation room with a massage table. My past and present were colliding like two particles in the Large Hadron Collider. It felt just plain weird.

I kept my inner freak-out to myself as I set up. And once I started presenting, I quickly fell into the easy flow of teaching what I love. At the start of the presentation, I asked participants to rate their general stress levels, and to raise their hands when I called out the level that best described how they felt. Every employee put up their hand for moderate to severe stress.

The workshop topic was on finding balance and included several reflexology points specific to stress—some of which you're going to learn shortly. After I showed participants how to locate their reflexology points, they were busy massaging their feet with their thumbs and knuckles.

At the end of the workshop, I asked if anyone was interested in experiencing what a reflexology stick felt like. Almost every hand in the room shot up in the air. People lined up at the front of the classroom, and one after another hopped up on the massage table for me to test their Kidney, adrenal, and Liver reflexology points. It was surprising how consistently sensitive everyone's feet were. I'd never seen so many people flinch with such a gentle touch of the stick.

Out of over a dozen employees, only one had what I considered to be a normal level of sensitivity for a new client. Everyone else had extremely sensitive reflexology points at levels consistent with what I would expect to see in someone with a long-standing, chronic health condition.

Based on their sensitivity levels, I could see the writing on the wall for health problems down the road. Most of the people shrugged off the seriousness with a nervous laugh. They remarked that they were indeed stressed and in need of a break, but they didn't have the time to do anything about it.

Please don't let this be you. It is so much easier to turn things around at the energy level before health issues show up in the body. So *please* pay close attention to the points in this chapter because your feet will let you know when it's time to take a step back and relax. Let's start with your number one stress indicator—the Liver point.

Chinese Reflexology Point for the Liver

Of all the energy meridians and organs in your body, the Liver is the one that is most impacted by stress. Liver disharmonies affect your entire body because no other organ has a greater influence on the flow of qi in your body than the Liver.

One of the Liver's key TCM functions is to ensure that your qi is flowing smoothly. However, when you're under stress, this can cause your Liver qi to stagnate, which adversely affects the flow of qi throughout your body.

When your Liver is out of balance, it can make you feel even more susceptible to stress. Proper flowing qi is necessary for health, vitality, and well-being, so it's essential to address Liver imbalances in order to restore your mental, emotional, and physical states of equilibrium. Let's take a closer look at this organ and energy meridian.

What Your Liver Does

The liver is one of the largest organs in your body. It's located on the right side of your body below the diaphragm. This organ is shaped like an upside-down right triangle. What's that? You've forgotten your geometry? A right triangle has one corner that is a perfect 90-degree angle. So the liver's shape resembles the sail of a sailboat, only turned sideways with the longer edge parallel to the horizon.

The liver has many functions. These include filtering toxins from the blood, regulating blood glucose levels, storing vitamins and minerals, and producing bile, which helps break down fats during the digestive process.

What Your Liver Does According to Traditional Chinese Medicine

One of the Liver's primary roles is to ensure the smooth flow of qi throughout the entire body. However, the Liver is susceptible to emotions such as anger and frustration. Stress also has a huge impact on the health of the Liver. When you're full of tension, the flow of qi is adversely affected and your Liver reflexology point becomes extremely sensitive.

If qi is not flowing smoothly, it can become congested and generate heat. This is like throwing a wrench into the gears of an engine. If the gears can't move, the engine begins to overheat. The same thing can happen in your body when Liver qi is not flowing smoothly. It can turn into a condition known as *Liver fire*, where the Liver drives qi upward to your head, resulting in migraines, irritability, or a red face. It is a literal manifestation of being hotheaded.

Congested qi in the Liver can also disturb neighboring organs. There's a condition in Chinese Medicine referred to as the *Liver attacking the Spleen*. What this means is that when Liver qi is congested, it can disturb the Spleen and Stomach, which then negatively affects your digestion.

The Liver also plays an important role in storing blood and regulating the amount of blood flowing into the body. When you're exercising, the Liver releases blood to your arms and legs. When you're at rest, the Liver draws the blood back in for storage.

Because of this close relationship between the Liver and blood, if there is not enough blood in the body, this results in the zang fu pattern (energy meridian disharmony) known as *Liver blood deficiency*. This has far-reaching effects and can affect vision; menstrual periods; sleep; emotions; and the tendons, ligaments, and cartilage in the body.

How to Locate Your Liver Point

The Liver point is located on the sole of the right foot. You'll find it next to the Kidney point in the top left quadrant of the right sole. After all that talk about the liver being shaped like a triangle, it's rather ironic that its reflexology point is actually shaped like a square. The Liver point extends from the Kidney point toward the outer edge of the foot. It includes the area below the ball of foot and above the horizontal line dividing the foot in half.

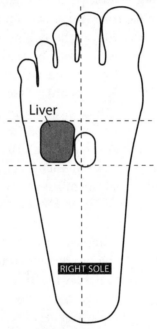

Chinese Reflexology Liver Point

How to Massage Your Liver Point

IMPORTANT

Because the liver is a large organ that filters blood, it can be a vessel for holding toxins in your body. It is important that you massage the Liver point only if you are consistently massaging all of the other points you've learned so far—especially the points for the Kidneys, Bladder, and lymphatic drainage. These other points help your body to clear away toxins more efficiently.

If you massage all of the points in this book as directed, it is very unlikely that you will experience detox symptoms (see Chapter 7). Instead, you will be very gently supporting your body to clear out toxins at a rate it can manage.

Use your thumbs to massage the Liver point in an up and down direction, where up is toward your toes and down is toward your heel. Because the reflexology area is so large, you can also reach the fingers of both hands around your right foot, and then use both thumbs to press into the point and massage in small circles. Begin at the top of the Liver point and work your way across and down.

Alternately, you can use the knuckle of your index finger to massage the point in an up and down motion, or press into a sensitive point more deeply. Apply a thin layer of lubricant such as massage oil or lotion to the reflexology point if you are using your knuckle. Because it is such a large area to massage, you'll want to reduce friction so that the skin on your knuckle does not become irritated. If your knuckle starts to feel a little sensitive, use your thumb instead.

After you finish massaging the point, grab a tissue or paper towel and wipe off any excess oil or lotion. You don't want to have such a big slippery square on your foot if you're walking on a smooth surface afterward.

Regardless of whether you use your thumbs or knuckles, massage this point for a maximum of 15 seconds. You can increase the time up to 30 seconds, but before you do, you should be practicing *all* of the reflexology points you've learned to date at least twice a week. The Putting It All Together chapter will give you direction on how to increase the massage time for reflexology points.

If you've been dealing with chronic stress for a long time, you can expect to have a very sensitive Liver point. The point may also feel hard and dense to the touch, like you're pressing on a piece of rubbery tire. During periods of high stress, the sensitivity for this point will noticeably increase.

Chinese Reflexology Point for the Adrenal Glands

In poker, there's something called a *tell*. This is a movement or change in behavior that gives other players a clue about the cards you're holding. For example, a person may lean forward or place their chips down more forcefully when they believe they have a weak hand. They're bluffing and posturing, but their tell gives them away.

You have a tell on your foot. Well actually, all of the Chinese reflexology points on your feet are tells, but there's one point that lets you know if you're deceiving yourself.

Have you ever answered, "I'm fine," when someone asks how you're doing? It's almost a reflexive response. If someone greets you with, "How's it going?" you automatically answer, "Good," even if things aren't so good. I know I've done it millions of times. Okay, maybe hundreds. My six-year-old son would say it's impossible to say something *millions* of times.

So I'll ask my clients how things are going or how work is, and they'll usually say that things are good. However, when I feel the tell on their foot, I know otherwise. So, what's the tell? I'll tell you.

It is the Chinese reflexology point for the adrenal gland. As soon as I press into this point, if someone has had a really crappy and stressful week, I'll instantly know. The adrenal gland point becomes hypersensitive when a person is going through a period of high stress. Often, I'll press the tip of the reflexology stick into the adrenal gland point and my client will flinch and yelp, "What was *that* point?"

The stakes are high because this point lets you know when stress levels are affecting your body. The adrenal gland point doesn't let you lie to yourself. So even if you think you're practicing enough self-care and taking it easy during a stressful period, this point will tell you the truth.

As you massage your feet regularly, you'll get a sense of the baseline sensitivity for your adrenal gland point. Over time, with regular and consistent massage, the sensitivity will decrease. However, during periods of high stress, the sensitivity levels for this point will immediately and dramatically spike upward. This lets you know that you are affecting the flow of qi in your body, and it's time to take a step back and let go of the stress as best you can.

I had my own wake-up call when we were selling our home. My husband and I thought we had planned everything perfectly in terms of timing. We worked out a target sale date so that we could move into a new home in time to register my son for the next school year.

However, we hadn't counted on the San Francisco Bay Area housing market going crazy, with selling prices soaring 10 to 15 percent over the asking prices, houses snapped up in a few days, and over a dozen offers per home. These conditions made it much more challenging for us to purchase a new home within the timeline we created.

We also forgot to factor in the 30-day period for close of escrow. This would delay our home hunting by almost a month, bringing us into the summer vacation months of traditionally low housing inventory.

After meeting with our real estate agent, we realized that we had to move up the target sale date of our house by a month. This gave us only a week to get our property ready for a weekend open house. Then our agent told us that it was common to do a broker tour on the Thursday before the weekend, so we had two fewer days to prepare. In order to list the home in time for the tour, we had to have the house ready for photos on Tuesday. Essentially, we had four days to get our lived-in home—with cat and kid—to show quality.

The days leading up to the open house were insane. I had multiple checklists for each room of the house with dozens of action items ranging from *polish the granite counters* for the kitchen to *install patio stones* for the backyard. It was an intense and highly stressful period for me.

I was so busy chugging my way through the checklists that I started worrying about how I would get everything done in time. Then, about halfway through the week, I noticed a slight ache in my feet. Most people ignore minor discomfort in their feet. If I feel anything unusual in my feet, however, I immediately pay attention.

When I sat down to massage my feet, I noticed that the reflexology points for my adrenal glands and Spleen were way more sensitive than usual. Remember how worrying too much is bad for the Spleen? I knew the sore point was a sign that I was fretting too much about the house.

On top of that, my adrenal gland point went from its usual sensitivity level of zero to a three. This let me know that the stress and worry were affecting my body. Receiving immediate feedback from my reflexology points reminded me to relax and scale back my to-do list.

Whether or not I polished the kitchen counter wouldn't change someone's mind about buying the house. I also had to remind myself that the Universe was looking out for me and to surrender to whatever happened. This enabled me to stop being so serious and take a more lackadaisical approach. I got the main things done, but I cut back on things that didn't need to be perfect.

Ironically, during the first day of the open house, a hand towel sat in plain view on the living room shelf. I had spent a lot of time arranging the books so that they were color-coordinated with the room. To make the shelf picture perfect, I learned the art of book stacking—did you know that there are seven different ways to stack books? Anyhow, I had accidentally left the new hand towel for the bathroom in a messy pile on the bookshelf.

And you know what? It didn't matter because our house sold in less than a week. It was a good lesson for me. All of those things that you worry about often don't really matter in the end.

Thankfully, my reflexology points were like a best friend reminding me to chill out and that everything would work out for the best. Because the adrenal gland point is so responsive to stress, it can be your best friend, too, reminding you to take a deep breath and relax. So take a deep breath right now and I'll tell you more about this BFF point.

What Your Adrenal Glands Do

The adrenal glands are shaped like pyramids and they sit on top of your kidneys. You've got two adrenal glands in total, one above each kidney. These glands secrete hormones that influence and regulate blood pressure and metabolism. They also secrete cortisol, which helps to reduce inflammation in the body.

The adrenal glands are probably best known for releasing adrenaline. That's the hormone that triggers the fight or flight response in your body. Adrenaline speeds up your heart rate and increases blood flow to your muscles so that you're ready to either beat the crap out of someone or run for your life. Of course, as we go about our day, we don't usually encounter life-or-death situations. So instead of burning off the adrenaline-induced energy, our bodies are left in a state of heightened stress, pulling us off-balance both physically and mentally.

How to Locate Your Adrenal Gland Point

The reflexology points for the adrenal glands are located on the soles of your feet above your Kidney points. The adrenal gland point on your right foot corresponds to the gland on the right side of the body, and the point on your left foot is for the left side of your body.

To locate this point, you'll use your Kidney point as a guide. Let's start with the left foot as an example. Find your Kidney point on your left sole, where two-thirds of the point is located in the top left quadrant and the other third in the top right.

Once you've located your Kidney point, imagine a vertical line dividing this point in half. Where this line intersects the top of the Kidney point is where you'll find the adrenal gland point. It's a small circle that slightly overlaps the Kidney point. Looking at the diagram, you'll see that the outline for these two points looks like an elongated pearl hoop earring turned upside down.

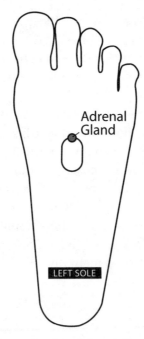

Chinese Reflexology Adrenal Gland Point

How to Massage Your Adrenal Gland Point

To massage your adrenal gland point, use the knuckle of your index finger to press firmly into this point while twisting at the same time. You'll apply the same twisting motion as you did for the solar plexus point, where your wrist turns back and forth as if you were jiggling a key in a door lock, or grasping onto a doorknob and rattling it. Massage this point for a maximum of 15 seconds per foot.

Chinese Reflexology Point for the Pituitary Gland

When it comes to maintaining balance in your body, the endocrine system plays a critical role. This system is a network of glands that produce and secrete hormones for regulating different functions in the body, including blood pressure, metabolism, growth, and reproduction. Your pituitary gland is the head honcho of the endocrine system. So if you want to be in balance, this gland needs to function properly in order to support your body in maintaining its natural equilibrium.

What Your Pituitary Gland Does

The pituitary gland is a pea-sized gland located at the base of the brain. Don't let its small size fool you, because this gland packs a powerful punch. It is considered to be the master gland of your endocrine system because it produces hormones that stimulate the production of hormones in other endocrine glands. The pituitary gland is like the conductor of an orchestra, directing the individual musicians to play together to produce a harmonious symphony, or in this case, a harmonious body.

How to Locate Your Pituitary Gland Point

The pituitary gland point is easy to find. It's a small circle located in the middle of the big toe pad, but it's slightly closer to the inside edge of the foot. You have a pituitary gland point on each big toe.

To fine-tune your location of this point, check for where you feel the most sensitivity in the middle of your toe pad. Support the top of the toe with the same side hand. Then press deeply onto the toe pad using your index finger knuckle from the opposite hand. Move the knuckle in tiny increments; where the point feels most sensitive is your pituitary gland point.

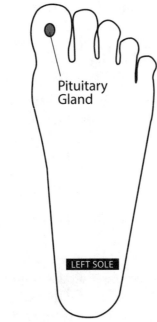

Chinese Reflexology Pituitary Gland Point

How to Massage Your Pituitary Gland Point

To massage this point, use the same technique that you applied for your adrenal gland point. Simply take the knuckle of your index finger and press it into the center of your big toe pad. After you've fine-tuned the positioning of your knuckle, massage with a twisting action for a total of 15 seconds per foot.

Points to Remember

After learning how to massage the points discussed in this chapter, you may be tempted to go to a yoga class or book an appointment at the spa. If that's what your reflexology points are telling you, then go for it. And for all those days in between yoga classes or spa appointments, remember to massage your reflexology points regularly. Here's a summary of these points.

1. Liver Point

- **Benefits:** supports Liver function to ensure the smooth flow of qi throughout the body, helps release effects of stress

- **Location:** square on the sole of the right foot in the top left quadrant; left of the Kidney point, below the ball of the foot, and above the horizontal halfway line

- **Massage Technique:** massage up and down (toe to heel direction) with thumb or knuckle; apply lubricant if using knuckle to massage

- **Recommended Time:** 15 seconds (can increase to 30 seconds after practicing reflexology regularly for several weeks)

2. Adrenal Gland Point

- **Benefits:** harmonizes adrenal glands and provides a warning that stress levels are too high

- **Location:** on the soles of both feet; small circle on top of the Kidney point

- **Massage Technique:** press and twist with knuckle
- **Recommended Time:** 15 seconds per foot

3. Pituitary Gland Point

- **Benefits:** "master gland" for endocrine system for balancing body's hormones
- **Location:** small circle in the center of the big toe pad (slightly closer to the inside edge of the foot) of both feet
- **Massage Technique:** press and twist with knuckle
- **Recommended Time:** 15 seconds per foot

CHAPTER 12

EMBRACING CHANGE

LARGE INTESTINE, LUNG, AND GALL BLADDER POINTS

Embracing change allows you to transform your health and your entire existence. However, it's not always easy to change, especially when your mind resists. When you're feeling stuck in life, your qi can also become stuck. This creates a self-perpetuating cycle where the stuck energy affects your physical body as well as your mental and emotional states. This, in turn, affects your ability to take action, and then you feel even more stuck and the cycle continues.

The great thing about a self-perpetuating cycle that involves qi is that *you can use energy to break the cycle.* Sometimes all it takes is a little nudge to become unstuck. If you want to change your health and life, but just can't seem to get started or keep the momentum going, there are some powerful Chinese reflexology points that may be just what you need.

The three points that you'll learn in this chapter address energy imbalances that may be holding you back from embracing change. The Large Intestine point relates to the energy of letting go of the past. The Lung point is about releasing sorrow so that you can welcome new experiences and breathe in life. Finally, the Gall Bladder point is about choosing boldly and courageously to take action so that you follow through on your initiative.

When you shift the energy within, you shift the energy in your outer world, too. You start to see changes in your circumstances because of the changes you make in your approach to life, and a new self-perpetuating cycle begins, only this one is pretty darn awesome.

A Story of Letting Go: The Love of My Life

One of the best examples of a person who shifted his inner energy to heal his body is someone very close to my heart—my husband. In his early 20s, Zunaid appeared to be in the prime of his life. He was a distance runner, worked out regularly, and also trained in martial arts.

Then he went through hell and back again. He had ended a relationship with a woman he thought he would one day marry. She wanted to start a family right away, but he wasn't ready, so they broke up.

Zunaid was distraught and heartbroken. He went through a period of extreme stress lasting for several months. One day, he keeled over on the bathroom floor in excruciating pain with his pants around his ankles. The toilet bowl was filled with blood.

Zunaid was diagnosed with ulcerative colitis, a chronic condition with no medical cure other than the removal of his colon. His symptoms included persistent diarrhea, abdominal pain, and blood in his stool. He was prescribed medication that had many side effects, including headaches, loss of appetite, and muscle and joint pain. He couldn't eat properly, lost a lot of weight, and felt mentally and physically exhausted. As a result, he became reclusive and avoided seeing friends and leaving the house as much as possible.

After months of this isolated existence, Zunaid finally reached a breaking point. He put away the bottle of pills and made the conscious decision to heal himself. He meditated for two days straight, and after this intense period of self-reflection, his symptoms disappeared over the course of a few weeks. He never took the pills again.

For the next 20 years of his life, he was pretty much symptom-free and could eat whatever he wanted, including lots of pumpkin pie (his favorite food). During an annual checkup close to his 40th birthday, Zunaid was advised to get a colonoscopy because of the increased risk of colon cancer associated with his history of ulcerative colitis. He debated about whether to get this invasive procedure, but finally decided to do it for peace of mind. He scheduled an appointment with one of the foremost experts in inflammatory bowel disease who had performed hundreds of colonoscopies.

Zunaid was always very good about consistently massaging his own reflexology points, so I showed him how to rub the points for his Large Intestine to help release any physical, mental, or energetic remnants of the disease. Because he's my husband, he also has his own reflexology stick. In the weeks leading up to his colon procedure, he massaged the Large Intestine points on both of his feet every day.

Two weeks after the colonoscopy, he got his test results back. The doctor was astounded. She had never seen a case like his before—there was *no trace* of the disease in his colon. She told him that in every case prior to his, she could tell from the biopsy that there was a pre-existing condition. But for Zunaid, if she hadn't seen his medical history (he brought in a copy of his original diagnosis), she would never have known that he previously had colitis.

Immediately after telling him that his colon looked 100 percent normal, she then warned him of numerous dangers and advised that he see her regularly because even though he was in "remission," the disease could strike at any time. She did concede that he was a "good" patient, so instead of an annual visit, he could check in every 18 months. Zunaid and I had a good chuckle over this. We figured that she was probably baffled by his case and recited her warnings on autopilot.

So what made his colon completely free from any signs of colitis? Was it the meditation, lifestyle change, shift in attitude, or Chinese reflexology? I know that many overthinkers like to analyze their progress and even go so far as to break down the contribution of each healing modality by percentages. My husband said he did the same thing. With so many ways available to heal himself, he wanted to know which was most effective.

But then he came up with some very wise words, so I'll quote what he said: "It doesn't matter which is more effective, or how much each is contributing to your healing. What matters is that you're getting better."

Of course, I'm partial to believing that the reflexology played an integral role. However, that's the beauty of Chinese reflexology. It is a healing modality that is complementary with other therapies because it supports your body's natural healing process.

Chinese Reflexology Point for the Large Intestine

When Zunaid's relationship with the woman he thought he would marry ended (lucky for me), that's when the ulcerative colitis struck. The resulting distress and emotional upheaval manifested in his colon. Since the Large Intestine is associated with the energy of letting go, Zunaid had to release the past and also let go of what his life had become in order to embrace change and heal himself.

If you are holding on to the past, you may be creating your own energetic constipation. Massaging the Chinese reflexology point for the Large Intestine is a powerful way to begin the process of releasing stuck energy. Before we get into how to do this, let's look at how the large intestine fits in with the rest of your digestive system.

What Your Large Intestine Does

After the small intestine absorbs nutrients from chyme (if you forget what chyme is, take a quick peek at the section about the stomach in Chapter 10), the remaining undigested food travels to the large intestine.

We interrupt this anatomy lesson to bring you some excitement. I may be exaggerating slightly about the cheap thrills, but I do have two bits of trivia that could one day win you the grand prize in a cheesy game show. Now that would be exciting!

Trivia Item #1: Did you know that in an average adult, the large intestine is about five feet long? This is significantly shorter than the small intestine (about 20 feet), so you may be wondering why it is called the *large* intestine. It's because its diameter is wider than that of the small intestine.

Trivia Item #2: The large intestine is also referred to as the colon. It can be categorized into different sections, which include the cecum, ascending colon, transverse colon, descending colon, sigmoid colon, rectum, and anus. Yup, that's a lot of parts, and it's partly (bad pun intended) why there are so many Chinese reflexology points for the digestive system. Each section of the large intestine has its own reflexology point.

We now return to our regular anatomy and physiology lesson . . .

The large intestine absorbs vitamins that are produced by bacteria in the gut. It also absorbs water from chyme to form feces.

Bonus Trivia: Feces is also referred to as excrement, stool, turd, logs, poo, poop, and dingleberry. However, dingleberry only applies if it's still hanging on to your pet's butt. For example, "When my cat runs out of his litter box too quickly, I often find a *dingleberry,* and then I say a word that is a synonym for feces and also rhymes with sit."

What Your Large Intestine Does
According to Chinese Medicine

The role of the Large Intestine in Chinese Medicine is similar to its Western function in that it receives digested food matter from the Small Intestine. The Large Intestine then absorbs water from this matter and transforms it into feces.

It also influences our ability to let go of things—both physically and emotionally. While the Large Intestine literally releases waste from our body, it also reflects how easily we let go of the past. In order to choose change, we have to let go of our mental and emotional "waste" so that we can move forward.

How to Locate Your Large Intestine Point

This reflexology point consists of several points, each representing a different part of the large intestine. It is absolutely critical that these points be massaged in the correct sequence and direction. The points mirror the shape of the large intestine in the body, so it's important to follow the correct flow of qi because this follows the direction that chyme is passed through the colon.

The Large Intestine points on your feet are long and skinny and require strong pressure, making them difficult to adequately massage using just your fingers or knuckles. It's best to use a reflexology stick to stimulate these points.

However, there is another part of your body that you can massage instead of your feet. It's the Large Intestine reflexology area on your left hand. Just like your feet, the hands contain reflexology points for your body. The location of the points on your hand map out quite similarly to those on your feet.

For example, your big toe is where the brain point is on your foot, and your thumb is where this point is located on your hand. Likewise, the location of the Large Intestine point on your hand is similar to your foot.

While hand points can be more convenient to massage, they're not as powerful as the points on your feet. The foot reflexology points are the master control points for balancing energy in your meridians. It's also much easier to measure sensitivity levels in your feet than in your hands.

There are, however, times when it is simply not convenient to take off your shoes and rub your feet (oh, say while you're in the middle of a meeting at work). That's why it's "handy" to have a backup plan. So, let's take a look at your left hand.

This point is quite practical because you can use it when you're sitting on the toilet and need to do your business. After all, if you're on the toilet, you certainly don't want to be reaching down to rub your foot.

If you ever suffer from temporary constipation, you can massage this point to help get your qi flowing, which in turn helps get your poo flowing. Ew, that's gross, isn't it? My husband always tells me that I talk about bodily functions in inappropriate ways at inappropriate times, such as at the dinner table.

Just to be clear, this is for *temporary* constipation that may be due to one of the following reasons:

- You're feeling self-conscious because someone might hear you.

- The toilet or restroom is disgusting.

- You're in a rush and you have a limited amount of time to finish.

- All of the above.

The Large Intestine reflexology point on your left hand includes three points—the transverse colon, descending colon, and sigmoid colon. While there are also Large Intestine points on the right hand, we'll focus on the left hand only because this covers the end portion of the large intestine where the poo comes out. You're also going to learn a bonus point for the rectum and anus.

When I do an initial consultation with clients, I walk them through the energy imbalances on their feet, point by point. I always have to suppress a smile when I tell them, "That's your anus point." (Yes, I can be rather immature, in case you didn't already gather that from my dingleberry reference. I worked in the Internet industry at a time when 80 percent of my co-workers were men in their 20s. The office was always filled with music blasting and the bantering of toilet humor, so I was pretty good at letting them rip, too. Jokes, that is.)

The reflexology point for the transverse colon is a horizontal line located about halfway down the height of your palm. Continuing along, the descending colon is a vertical line along the outer edge of your palm directly below your baby finger. It begins at the end of the transverse colon point and descends downward to about one thumb width above your wrist crease.

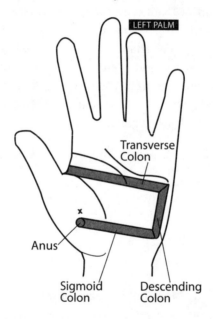

Chinese Reflexology Large Intestine Points on Hand

Finally, the sigmoid colon reflexology point is a horizontal line going from the descending colon to the thenar of your thumb. That's the big fleshy pad of your thumb that makes up part of your palm, which you learned about when you located the Stomach point.

Let's not forget the bonus point for the rectum and anus. You can find this point at the end of the sigmoid colon point. It's a small circle located just below the center of your thenar. If you imagine a point right in the middle of the big fleshy pad of your thumb (see the *x* on the diagram), the anus reflexology point is located just below it.

Remember how I compared different organs in the digestive system to different parts of a car? Well, I hope you enjoyed the auto analogies, because I have one more to share with you, courtesy of my husband. I told him how I was using car analogies to describe parts of the digestive system. I explained how the solar plexus was the onboard computer, the Spleen was the engine, and the Stomach was the gas tank.

Then my husband came up with his own comparison. He gleefully announced, "So the anus is the tail pipe!" His proclamation was accompanied by a tilt of his bum and a simulated toot sound. Yes, it was a proud moment for him.

How to Massage Your Large Intestine Point

Although there are different Large Intestine points on your hand, you can massage them together in one continuous motion. But first, I'll walk you through each point individually. Let's begin with the transverse colon located on your left palm. To massage this point, make a fist with your right hand and use your knuckles to stroke horizontally across your palm from *left* to *right*.

When you finish the stroke, pick up your knuckles, place them back at the left edge of your palm, and repeat. Massage for 15 strokes. It is important that you massage the transverse colon from left to right—going from the index finger toward the pinky—as this follows the flow of chyme through this portion of your colon.

To massage the descending colon point, use a single knuckle. I like to use the knuckle on the middle finger of my right hand to stroke the descending colon in a downward direction. Start at where the transverse colon ends and stroke in a *downward direction*, going from below your pinkie finger toward your wrist, until you reach the point where the sigmoid colon begins. When you finish the stroke, pick up your knuckle, place it back at the top of the descending colon point, and repeat. Do this for 15 strokes.

Finally, you'll use all four of your knuckles to massage the sigmoid colon point. Stroke horizontally from *right* to *left*, going from the outer edge of your palm toward the thumb. Do this also for 15 strokes.

When you are feeling confident and comfortable with locating these points, you can massage them all together as one continuous stroke. Start with the transverse colon and continue until you reach the end of the sigmoid colon. Massage all three points in one motion 15 times. An easy way to visualize the correct direction is to follow a clockwise motion when you are looking directly at your left palm.

To massage your rectum and anus point, use the knuckle of your right index finger. Press into the point and twist back and forth. Do this for about 15 seconds.

If you're massaging these points for temporary constipation, you'll want to take a breath and relax the muscles in your abdomen for a few seconds in order to release any tension that may be making you temporarily constipated. Then massage the intestinal points for another 15 strokes. Follow up with 15 seconds for the rectum and anus point. You'll be surprised at how much easier and quicker the poo comes out. My friends, who shall remain unnamed, always discreetly tell me that this routine works like a charm.

Chinese Reflexology Point for the Lungs

In addition to letting go of the past, Zunaid also had to release the sorrow he felt about his failed relationship because this was affecting his Lung meridian. In Chinese Medicine, the Lung and Large Intestine channels have a special relationship. When everything is working harmoniously, Lung qi descends, and this downward action helps to keep things moving through the Large Intestine. If Lung qi is weak, this can affect the function of the Large Intestine as there is not enough energy to properly move stuff through the colon, and this can lead to constipation or abdominal pain.

Massaging the reflexology points for both the Lungs and Large Intestine can help strengthen these two energy meridians. Aside from the physical benefit of keeping things moving smoothly, these two points can also help you break free from your past so that you can embrace new experiences and fully breathe in life.

What Your Lungs Do

The lungs are a pair of cone-shaped organs located in your chest. Air flows into your lungs through your windpipe, which then divides into two bronchi, one for each lung. From the bronchi, smaller tubes called bronchioles branch out through your lungs. The smallest tubes are surrounded by clusters of alveoli, which are tiny air sacs where the exchange of oxygen and carbon dioxide occurs.

The whole system looks like an upside-down tree where the windpipe is the tree trunk and the bronchi are where the trunk splits into two main branches. The bronchioles are smaller branches and twigs, and the alveoli are like leaves. Imagine wrapping all these branches with two oversized pink balloons—one for each lung—and you've got a vision of what's going on inside your chest.

What Your Lungs Do According to Traditional Chinese Medicine

It is said that the *Lungs govern qi and respiration*. This encompasses the Western medicine perspective of respiration, but with an added twist. The Lungs extract qi from the air and combine it with the qi that you get from food (gu qi) to produce another type of qi called *zong qi*. This qi supports the Heart and Lungs in carrying out their functions.

Honestly, there are so many different types of qi in Chinese Medicine that it can get quite complicated and confusing. Suffice it to say, all of it is good qi and all of it is needed for a healthy functioning body.

While we're on the topic of qi, however, there is one more that relates to the Lungs—it's called *wei qi*, also known as *defensive qi*. The Lungs help disperse wei qi to the skin, where it forms a barrier to protect the body against external evil (aka germs). Thus, the Lungs play an important role in keeping you healthy so that you can avoid catching a cold.

If you ever do find yourself on the verge of catching a cold or needing to get over one quickly, you'll find a cold remedy mini reflexology routine in the Resources section at the end of this book. This five-minute reflexology routine works like a charm. I've heard from readers all over the world about how it's helped them clear snotty noses, ease sore throats, and vanquish chest congestion.

The Lungs are also associated with the emotion of sadness. Grief is kryptonite for the Lungs. You only have to observe a person balled up in sorrow to see that their hunched posture compresses the chest and disrupts the flow of qi through their Lungs.

Massaging the Lung reflexology point can help strengthen Lung qi and restore the proper flow of energy. As your Lung qi improves, don't be surprised if your energy levels increase and your ability to breathe in life and new experiences also becomes easier.

How to Locate Your Lung Point

The Lung point is located on the soles of your feet. It's a rectangular-shaped area on the ball of the foot below the three middle toes. The top portion of this point corresponds to the upper part of the lungs and the bottom portion of the reflexology point corresponds to the lower part of the lungs. In addition, the right foot is for your right lung, and the left foot is for your left lung.

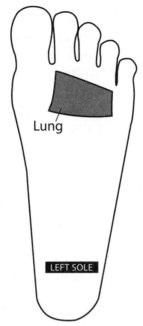

Chinese Reflexology Lung Point

How to Massage Your Lung Point

Because the reflexology area is so big, you can use two thumbs to massage it. Reach the fingers of both hands around your foot to provide support. Then press the thumbs into your Lung point, beginning in the top left corner. Massage in small circles for a couple of seconds, and then work your way across and down the entire reflexology area. Massage for 30 to 60 seconds per foot.

Chinese Reflexology Point for the Gall Bladder

If you recall, your adrenal gland point can tell you a lot about the stress levels in your life. The Gall Bladder point is equally revealing. When I massage this point on a client, I can learn a lot about their decision-making process. If the Gall Bladder point is very sensitive, I know that a client may be vacillating over a major life decision.

John was a classic case of weak Gall Bladder qi. The first time I massaged his Gall Bladder point, I was struck by how defined it was on his foot. I could trace the outline of the point with the reflexology stick. It reminded me of running a finger over an embossed logo on a business card.

When I asked John whether he found it challenging to make decisions, he shared that he'd been debating for a year whether or not to stay in a relationship. He also laughed when I asked if he had trouble deciding what to order off a menu, because that described him perfectly.

In short, your Gall Bladder can say so much about your ability to make a decision. Read on to learn more . . . if you choose.

What Your Gallbladder Does

The gallbladder is a small, pear-shaped sac located behind and below your liver. The main function of the gallbladder is to store and concentrate bile produced by the liver. After you chow down on a greasy diner breakfast, your gallbladder releases bile into your duodenum—the first section of the small intestine—to help digest the fat from your meal.

What Your Gall Bladder Does
According to Traditional Chinese Medicine

In Traditional Chinese Medicine, the Gall Bladder has a close relationship with the Liver. These two organs have a yin and yang relationship where they depend on each other in order to function properly. They both help support the sinews, which include connective tissue such as ligaments, tendons, and cartilage. The Liver nourishes the sinews with blood, while the Gall Bladder provides the supporting qi.

The Gall Bladder also stores bile produced by the Liver. This perspective is similar to the Western medical perspective. Where the views differ significantly is in the mental and emotional aspects of the organ.

It is said that the *Gall Bladder controls decisiveness.* What this means is that the Gall Bladder affects your ability to choose decisively. Being indecisive is associated with a weak Gall Bladder, whereas a healthy Gall Bladder provides the courage and initiative to help you make decisions.

While massaging your Gall Bladder point won't turn you into a decision-making pro overnight, it will help strengthen your Gall Bladder qi. Over time, this will help you to choose more decisively.

Indecision creates inaction, which stops you from moving forward. As you start making small choices more easily, such as ordering the rigatoni instead of the penne, you'll find that the big choices begin to feel easier, too.

How to Locate Your Gall Bladder Point

The Gall Bladder point is located on the sole of your right foot. You'll need to use your Liver point as a guide in order to find the Gall Bladder point. So let's do a quick refresher on where your Liver point is located. It's a square-shaped area on your right sole beside your Kidney point.

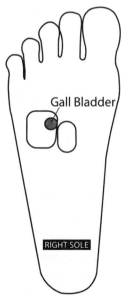

Chinese Reflexology Gall Bladder Point

The Gall Bladder point is a circle located in the top right quadrant of the Liver point. Its location varies slightly for each person. For some people, it will be higher on the Liver point, and for others it may be slightly lower. Use your thumb or knuckle to press in the top right quadrant. Move your thumb or knuckle in small increments to feel for the most sensitive area. Once you find it, you've found your Gall Bladder point.

As you become more proficient and comfortable with massaging your reflexology points, you'll get a better sense for exactly where your Gall Bladder point is located. This sense of knowing comes with practice.

How to Massage Your Gall Bladder Point

You can use either your thumb or index finger knuckle to press into this point. If you're using your thumb, lean in to the point with your body weight and massage using a small circular motion. If you're using your knuckle, simply press and twist. Massage for a total of 15 seconds.

Points to Remember

So now you know how important it is to let go of the past. You've learned some handy points, including the anus (tee-hee), to help you release the old and welcome the new. Here's a summary of what we covered in this chapter.

1. Large Intestine Point on Hand

- **Benefits:** supports Large Intestine function to keep things moving smoothly through the colon and helps with letting go of the past; helps clear energy blocks associated with temporary constipation

- **Location:** on the left palm; transverse colon is a horizontal line in the middle of the palm; descending colon is a vertical line along the outer edge of the palm below the baby finger; sigmoid colon is a horizontal line from the descending colon to the thenar of the thumb; rectum and anus is a small circle at the end of the sigmoid colon point

- **Massage Technique:** use knuckles to massage clockwise when facing the palm, beginning with the transverse colon; press and twist with knuckle for the rectum and anus point
- **Recommended Strokes:** 15 strokes in clockwise direction only, finishing with 15 seconds on the rectum and anus point

2. Lung Point

- **Benefits:** supports Lung function, assists descending action of Lung qi, helps to release effects of sadness and grief so that you can embrace life
- **Location:** on the soles of both feet, area on the ball of the foot below the three middle toes
- **Massage Technique:** use thumbs to press and massage in small circles, working your way across and down the point
- **Recommended Time:** 30 to 60 seconds per foot

3. Gall Bladder Point

- **Benefits:** supports Gall Bladder function to help with decisive decision-making
- **Location:** on the sole of the right foot, small circle in the top right quadrant of the Liver point
- **Massage Technique:** press and twist with knuckle or massage in a small circular motion with thumb
- **Recommended Time:** 15 seconds

CHAPTER 13

Moving Forward Fully Supported

Shoulder, Knee, Inner Hip, and Outer Hip Points

What am I resisting? is a great question to ask yourself if you have any knee, hip, ankle, or foot problems. Is there a change you want to make that you've been avoiding? Are you scared of making the "wrong" choice? Or are there so many options you don't know where to begin?

Fear is often at the root of feeling stuck in life. However, when you fail to take action when the moment presents itself, you're telling your body that you want to stay put. You don't want to move. So your body listens and helps you *not* move.

Hesitation, procrastination, and inertia can manifest as problems in the parts of your body that propel you forward—your legs, hips, knees, ankles, and feet. And if you don't feel supported when heading in a new direction, this can manifest as problems in your shoulders because you feel burdened and overwhelmed.

The reflexology points in this chapter can help you move forward when you're feeling stuck. The shoulder point lets you know if feeling unsupported is stopping your progress, so that you can then shift your thinking to lighten your load. Points for the knees and hips support movement and reflect how easily you step forward in life. More ease and flow in your joints results in more ease and flow in your qi, and subsequently more ease and flow in your thoughts and actions.

The Importance of Moving Forward

True healing is a journey into facing your fears—fear of the unknown, fear of things staying the same, fear of failure, and even fear of success. Don't be scared of jumping off the cliff. What you should be afraid of is sitting on the precipice and *not* moving. In order to move forward in life, you actually have to *do something*.

Of course, it's not always as easy as it sounds. Sometimes we think we're making great strides forward, and then *wham!* Fear stops us in our tracks. I can claim firsthand experience on this one—literally.

In my early 30s, I had an idea for a cooking show. This was at the dawn of the era of celebrity chefs, when most cooking shows were like watching a food demonstration at the supermarket. My idea was to make a fun and sexy cooking show featuring three fashionably dressed friends who would meet each week to cook a meal together. While sharing how to make the food with viewers, the hosts would also share tidbits and happenings from their lives—sort of like a cooking show/soap opera/reality TV show that promoted healthy and sumptuous meals.

My first plan of action was to find three hosts. I had one friend who was a total foodie. When she e-mailed me a picture of herself holding a roast on a platter, I thought, *there's my first host.* I had another friend who was really into acting and had appeared in some commercials. She couldn't cook, but she looked good on camera, so I figured I could write her inability to cook as part of the show. If she could make the recipe, anybody could.

That left me with finding one more host. As I pointed my finger in the air and mentally counted, *one, two . . . three* was pointing right back at me. At the time, I was really uncomfortable with putting myself out there. Being in front of the camera filled me with terror and self-consciousness. But as they say, the show must go on. I became the third host.

Without any television experience, we put together a demo and went to the Banff Television Festival to pitch our idea. It was a huge success, and we had five production companies vying to make a deal with us. We ended up signing with the company that had the highest rated cooking show in Canada at the time.

I returned home triumphant, and the wheels were in motion for creating a super fun and sexy show that would appeal to a broad audience and encourage people to eat better. Within days, my friends and I had our very first conference call with the executive producer at the production company. After the call, I was a nervous ball of energy.

I realized I was on the cusp of a *huge* life change, and the entire trajectory of my life was about to shift. We knew that the show's success hinged on the hosts being open and vulnerable, so essentially we had to share a lot of our personal stuff on TV. If there ever was a time for my mind to create resistance, this was it.

Sure enough, after I hung up the phone, I dashed out of my apartment and down the steps that I'd descended without incident hundreds of times before. Only this time I tripped on a crack, twisted my ankle, and went flying. Eventually, I managed to hobble back into my apartment and called a friend to take me to the doctor.

Throughout the ordeal, I couldn't help but notice how my fear of moving forward had manifested in a literal way. As a result of my sprained ankle, I couldn't move forward. I was on crutches for weeks.

I learned a very valuable lesson that day—to address the fear before it manifests in my body. Now if I ever notice a weird twinge in my knee or a funny feeling in my foot, the first thing I do is look at what is going on in my life and figure out where I am dragging my feet and rebelling against change.

(In case you're wondering what happened to the cooking show, I let various other fears stop me, and the whole thing sort of imploded. Had I continued moving forward despite being afraid, maybe you'd be seeing me on TV right now. Looking back, however, I see how even this "failure" was part of following my life's path. It gave me the confidence to make online videos on Chinese reflexology. *Psst,* you may still see me on television one day!)

Don't let fear stop *you.* Sometimes life changes are easier to make and feel less scary when you are supported along the way. So your first order of business is to create a support system for yourself, but look beyond leaning on just your friends and family. Remember that there is a powerful support network available to you at any time—the Universe. It is here to support your health and well-being. The Chinese reflexology point for the shoulder can also help support you, so let's move forward with this point.

Chinese Reflexology Point for the Shoulders

The shoulder point is awesome for muscle-related issues—everything from waking up with a funny crick in your shoulder to recovering from an old injury. I was fortunate to witness the power of this point early in my reflexology practice.

After I had been studying Chinese reflexology for a few months, my teacher, Dr. Gilbert Tay, asked students to bring a friend or family member to class. He jokingly referred to our guests as guinea pigs because they were volunteering to receive Chinese reflexology sessions.

Under Dr. Tay's close supervision, I worked with Martina, who was the girlfriend of one of the other students. Martina was bright and perky, but she had a really low tolerance for pain. As I massaged the Chinese reflexology point for her left shoulder, she grimaced even more than she had for the other points on her feet. When I asked her about it, she told me that she had slept funny the night before and had woken up with a pain in her shoulder.

I asked if she was willing to put up with a little more reflexology for her shoulder. Martina was a good sport and agreed, even though she was squirming uncomfortably as I massaged the point on her foot.

When it was over, she sighed in relief and lamented about how much the shoulder point had hurt. Midway through her sentence, she suddenly sat straight up and exclaimed, "Hey! The pain in my shoulder is gone!" Dr. Tay looked over and calmly pronounced, "Many miracles happen here."

It was the first time I had practiced Chinese reflexology on another person and witnessed a miracle. I felt indescribable joy. And now it is my pleasure to share this amazing point with you.

What Your Shoulders Do

Shoulders represent the burdens we carry in life. When you see a person with stooped shoulders, you know that they've been carrying a lot of energetic baggage and feel like they have the weight of the world resting on them.

If you've been feeling a little slouchy lately, it's time to dump some of that weight off your shoulders. Often overthinkers are overachievers because we want to do everything ourselves. We *think* no one else can do a task better than we can. However, this isn't about competency, it's about *control*. Hint: delegating is good.

When you feel weighted down, the reflexology point for the shoulders can remind you that you don't have to do everything yourself. You don't have to carry the load for the whole world. You don't even have to carry this burden for yourself, because you can always choose to lighten up.

As you massage your shoulder point, visualize healing energy flowing through your shoulders. As you do this, it will remind you that it's not just your energy flowing through your deltoids and trapezius muscles—the energy of the Universe is also there to support and revitalize you.

The shoulder is a ball-and-socket joint. If you've ever constructed an exosuit out of a popular brick-based building toy that my son loves, then you're familiar with this type of joint. One end has a ball and the other has a socket. On your body, the ball is the rounded end of your humerus (upper arm bone), and the socket is part of your scapula (shoulder blade).

Your shoulders have the widest range of motion of all the joints in your body. However, what they gain in mobility, they lose in stability. This makes the shoulders more prone to injury, strain, and overuse.

Your shoulders do so much to support you, so you can return the favor by massaging the Chinese reflexology points that support the flow of qi and blood through them.

How to Locate Your Shoulder Point

The shoulder point is located on the sole below the pinky toe, and it extends to the outside edge of the foot. The reflexology point for your right shoulder is on your right foot, and the point for your left shoulder is on the left foot. In addition, the area closest to the base of your pinky toe, near the outer edge of the foot, corresponds to the region where your shoulder meets your neck.

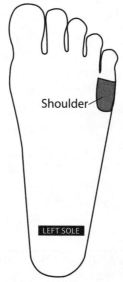

Chinese Reflexology Shoulder Point

How to Massage Your Shoulder Point

Place your thumb on the point and massage in an up and down direction, where up is toward your pinky toe, and down is toward your heel. Use a firm pressure like what you'd use to smooth out air bubbles when sticking down a sheet of shelf liner or contact paper. Be sure to press and massage on this point along the edge of the foot, too. Massage for 15 to 30 seconds per foot.

If any area feels extra sensitive or hard to the touch, press in more deeply and massage with small circles. The entire reflexology point may feel hard if you've had a previous shoulder injury. This is a different feeling from a callus, which you'll feel on the surface of the skin. The hardness that I'm referring to feels like a callus *under* the skin.

Chinese Reflexology Point for the Knees

Your knees enable you to step forward in life. Thus, if you're having problems with your knees, it's a good idea to look at where you may be stopping yourself from moving forward. If you have a sudden injury, there may be a new direction in your life that you are vehemently resisting.

If your knee problems are lingering and chronic, perhaps there is something that has been going on for a longer period of time. It could be a low-level concern in the back of your mind. However, it's always there under the surface, slowly wearing away at your body and your knees' ability to move easily and freely.

Or perhaps your mind is set in one direction, and your body is trying to remind you that your heart and soul want to take you in another direction. When you resist the flow of life and try to control it, that's when knee issues arise. Your body is simply trying to tell you something that your bullheaded mind is too stubborn to hear. Sometimes all it takes to kick-start the healing process is to be open-minded.

A few years ago when I was training for a triathlon, I joined an online runners group for moms. It was great to have a network of people to train with, but I couldn't help but notice the numerous posts from members with knee issues. As a result, I wrote an article on my blog about the Chinese reflexology point for the knees.

Even though the article was written for my local running group, it reached people all over the world. Six months after posting the article, I received a comment on my blog from a man living in Singapore. I've taken the liberty to paraphrase what he wrote because he used a lot of abbreviations:

> Your massage treatment for knee pain works! I've been having this knee pain for at least five years. Every time I bend or squat, I'll feel a sharp pain on the inner side of my right knee. I happened to chance upon your website, followed your technique, and it worked within a few minutes. I bend or squat, lo and behold, no pain, good as normal. So grateful to you for sharing this info . . . *a big thank you.*

His comment made my day and filled my heart with joy. This is what inspires me to write, teach, and share. The greatest abundance I receive isn't money—it is the joy I receive when I see someone use what they've learned to transform their life.

What Your Knees Do

The knee is the largest joint in your body. It connects your femur (thigh bone) to your tibia (shinbone) and patella (kneecap). Because the knee is such a complex joint, it is prone to overuse and injury, which can result in pain and inflammation.

In Chinese Medicine, stabbing pain in the knees is attributed to stagnant qi and blood through the area. Dull, achy pain, on the other hand, is due to a deficiency in the Kidneys. When the Kidneys are weak, they are unable to properly carry out their role of controlling the bones. The bones in the knees weaken, and this results in the achiness in the knees.

Massaging the Chinese reflexology point for the knees helps to restore the proper flow of qi and blood regardless of whether the pain is due to stagnation or deficiency. That's what is so great about Chinese reflexology. You don't have to figure out whether there is too much energy congested in an area or not enough flowing. Massage your points and your body will naturally do what it needs to.

How to Locate Your Knee Point

The Chinese reflexology point for the knee is located on the outer edge of your foot where the skin meets the sole. It's a circle with a diameter that is slightly wider than the width of your thumb. To locate this point, use a finger to feel along the edge of your foot, following the line where the skin meets the sole.

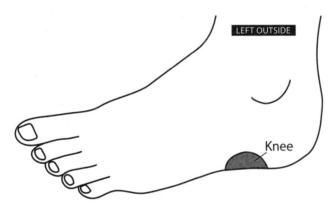

Chinese Reflexology Knee Point

Begin at your heel below your ankle and slide your finger forward toward your toes as you press with a medium pressure. Just past your heel, you'll feel a small depression along the side of your foot. This is where your knee point is located.

If you have any problems with your knees, the most tender spot will let you know that you've found your knee reflexology point. The left foot is for your left knee, and the right foot is for your right knee. You can measure your healing progress based on the sensitivity of the point. As you heal, the point will feel less sensitive.

How to Massage Your Knee Point

It can be a little awkward to reach the outer edge of your foot. I find the easiest way to reach this point is to stand on the floor and place your foot flat on the surface of a sturdy stool or chair, like you're stepping up on a stair. Then reach down with the same side hand and massage the point.

You can use either your thumb or the knuckle of your index finger to massage this point. If you're using your knuckle, apply lubricant to the point to avoid irritating the skin on your knuckle. Press and rub the reflexology area with a back and forth motion, going in the direction from toe to heel and back again. Massage each foot for 15 to 30 seconds.

If you have a knee injury, you can add extra massage time to support your body's healing process. After visiting your medical practitioner, follow their prescribed treatment and massage your knee point (on the injury side) for 60 seconds, three times a day until your knee is better. If you can't reach your foot because of the injury, enlist a friend or family member to rub the point for you.

For chronic knee pain, increase the massage times for both your knee and Kidney points. The Kidneys are important because of their role in controlling the bones. In Chinese Medicine, weak knees are associated with a deficiency in the Kidneys, so you'll need to massage your Kidney points to help strengthen this energy channel. Add an extra minute per day for both the knee and Kidney points on each of your feet.

Chinese Reflexology Points for the Hip

The hips bear the body's weight and enable us to walk, run, skip, dance, jump, and play. They support our bodies and carry us forward in life. When you consider the connection the hips have to moving forward in life, it gives new meaning to the expression *shooting from the hip.*

What Your Hips Do

The hip joint is a ball-and-socket joint just like your shoulder. As a result, it has quite a wide range of motion. In Chinese reflexology, there are actually two reflexology points for the hips. One is for the inner hip where your thighs come together, and the other point is for your outer hip where you'd place your hands if you were playing a game of Simon Says and Simon said to touch your hips.

How to Locate Your Inner Hip Point

The inner hip point is shaped like a curved breakfast sausage. To locate this reflexology point, place your thumb on the bony part of your inner ankle where it sticks out the most. Then slide your thumb off the ankle, toward the bottom of your foot, until you feel a slight depression just under the bone. Follow the curve below and behind the anklebone, and this is where the reflexology point for your inner hip is located. Your right foot is for the right inner hip, and your left foot is for the left side.

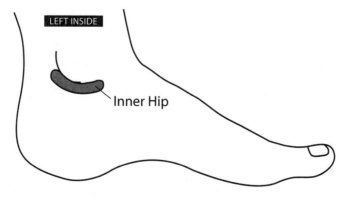

Chinese Reflexology Inner Hip Point

187

How to Massage Your Inner Hip Point

Let's start with your left foot. Apply some massage oil or lotion to the point. Then place your left thumb in the depression under the anklebone. Massage along the curve below the bone going from one end of the point to the other and back again. You're essentially rubbing this point back and forth. Do this for 15 to 30 seconds per foot.

Because there are nerves running through this area, you may feel a weird sensation when you massage this point if you accidentally hit a nerve. The sensation may feel like a mild electric shock, and it will vanish as quickly as it appeared. If this happens, use less pressure and massage for no more than 15 seconds in total.

How to Locate Your Outer Hip Point

The location of the outer hip point is very similar to the inner hip, only it is located on the outside of your foot. It is also shaped like a breakfast sausage that follows the curve of the anklebone.

To find this point on your foot, use your index finger to feel for a depression below the outer ankle. Then trace the curve of the ankle, below and behind the bone. The right foot is for the right outer hip, and the left foot is for the left side.

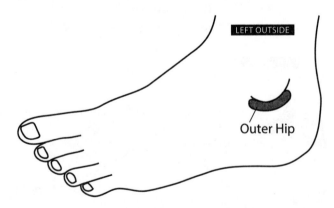

LEFT OUTSIDE

Outer Hip

Chinese Reflexology Outer Hip Point

How to Massage Your Outer Hip Point

To massage this reflexology point, you'll use the same technique that you used for the inner hip point. However, instead of using your thumb to rub the point, use your index finger. If you're massaging your left foot, use your left index finger. Remember to apply some massage oil or lotion to the point.

Press your finger into the depression under the anklebone. Then massage along the curve using a back and forth motion to cover the entire length of this point. Massage for 15 to 30 seconds per foot.

Just like with the inner hip point, there are a number of nerves close to the outer ankle so you may feel a weird sensation when you massage this point. If that's the case, ease up on the pressure you're applying and massage for only 15 seconds.

Points to Remember

So now you've got a handful (or should I say *foot-ful?*) of points to help you move forward with more ease and flow. Here's a summary of these four points for your joints.

1. Shoulder Point

- **Benefits:** improves qi and blood flow through the shoulder area and helps to release feelings of being overburdened
- **Location:** on soles of both feet, rectangular area under the pinky toe that extends to the outside edge of the foot
- **Massage Technique:** massage up and down (from toe to heel direction) with thumb
- **Recommended Time:** 15 to 30 seconds per foot

2. Knee Point

- **Benefits:** improves qi and blood flow through the knee joint and helps with moving forward in life
- **Location:** on the outside edge of both feet, in the depression above the heel where the skin meets the sole
- **Massage Technique:** massage back and forth (from toe to heel direction) with thumb or knuckle; apply lubricant if using knuckle to massage
- **Recommended Time:** 15 to 30 seconds per foot

3. Inner Hip Point

- **Benefits:** improves qi and blood flow through the inner hip joint and helps with moving forward in life
- **Location:** "breakfast sausage" on the inside edge of both feet, below and behind the anklebone
- **Massage Technique:** apply lubricant and massage back and forth with thumb
- **Recommended Time:** 15 to 30 seconds per foot

4. Outer Hip Point

- **Benefits:** improves qi and blood flow through the outer hip joint and helps with moving forward in life
- **Location:** "breakfast sausage" on the outside edge of both feet, below and behind the anklebone
- **Massage Technique:** apply lubricant and massage back and forth with index finger
- **Recommended Time:** 15 to 30 seconds per foot

CHAPTER 14

EXPRESSING YOUR BRILLIANCE

THROAT, OVARY, TESTICLE, UTERUS, AND PROSTATE POINTS

I've got a question for you—and it's a loaded one, but I know you're brave enough to answer it. Are you living your life purpose?

The reason I ask is because following your passion is directly related to your health and vitality. When you follow your soul's calling and use your talents and abilities to your highest potential, you're in the flow of life. You welcome in the revitalizing energy of the Universe and make choices that support your health and well-being.

No one ever sits down and consumes a full-sized bag of chips or an entire pint of ice cream in one sitting because they're high on life. On the other hand, when your life feels purposeful and fulfilled, you wake up so excited to greet the day that you're over-flowing with energy, happiness, and joy. And in this energetic space, you make choices that are good for your body.

The points in this chapter are extremely powerful for help-ing you express your brilliance and follow your soul's calling.

They include the throat point, as well as points for the reproductive system.

The throat point is related to the energy of speaking up and sharing your voice and ideas. The ovary, uterus, testicle, and prostate points are related to the energy of creation and making your mark on the world. All of these points can let you know when you're playing it safe, hiding in the background, or holding back on letting others (or yourself) know how amazing and brilliant you truly are.

I know that when you're feeling stuck in a job, relationship, or situation, it can seem almost impossible to walk away and follow your life purpose. That's a problem with our binary society. We feel it's all or nothing, but you merely have to look at a yin yang to be reminded that it doesn't have to be this way.

Yin and yang are not mutually exclusive. Even when one element is at its fullest, there is always a little bit of the other contained within. So no matter what your situation, there is a seed of your life purpose in it. All you need to do is nurture this seed for it to grow.

Since many people get stuck trying to figure out what their life purpose is, I've got a few tips to help you a little later in this book. For now, it's more important to plant the seed of possibility.

The Lowest Point in My Health

You've learned quite a bit about me in the stories I've shared in this book, but there's one more story I need to share with you. To be honest, I debated about whether or not to include it because it's so personal, and thus makes me feel very open and vulnerable. But since this chapter is about sharing your voice and expressing your brilliance, I certainly can't tell you to speak up if I hold back myself.

This is the story about what led me to Chinese reflexology and my firsthand experience of its healing powers. I've only told this to a few close friends and shared it with a small number of workshop participants, but now I'm going to share it with you. I should warn you, though—this is not a story for the squeamish.

After working in high tech for almost a decade and ignoring my soul's calling, my body finally got fed up with me. It started breaking down, and I experienced my year of illness, when I had one weird disease or health issue after another—everything from eye styes and a bladder infection that had me passing blood in my urine, to some strange ten-day splitting headache due to the meninges in my brain swelling, which by the way was never properly diagnosed, but in retrospect was most likely either viral meningitis or West Nile virus.

I felt like I was fading in and out of life like a translucent ghost on a TV show fading in and out of the scene. It got so bad that I wondered if I was dying, but the scary thing was that my life had become so meaningless that I didn't really care. Ironically, it was not caring that scared me into caring.

I hit rock bottom when I came down with the weirdest of all ailments in a body part that I had never heard of before. Here comes the part of the story that might make you feel a little squeamish.

There are two pea-sized glands located next to the vaginal opening. They're part of the reproductive system, and they're called Bartholin's glands. One of mine developed a cyst, which then became infected. At first, I wrote it off as either a pimple or boil. Then it got bigger.

The swelling seemed to go down after I slept, so in the morning I would still get up and go to work. After a few more days, the infected cyst got even bigger, more obtrusive, and very painful. I also felt a general sense of malaise throughout my entire body. The swelling grew to the size of a chicken egg.

Looking back, I don't know how I managed to ignore it for so long. I guess working in a high stress job enabled me to get so good at tuning out my body that I managed to tune out a giant swelling next to my sit bones.

When it became intolerable, I finally went to the hospital emergency room. The doctor had to lance the swelling and squeeze the pus out of it. I was left with a gaping abscess in my body, which the doctor stuffed with a trail of gauze.

When you have an abscess in your lady parts with a ribbon of gauze hanging out of it, you know you've reached a low point in your health. However, it motivated me to finally make changes in my life.

After months of Zunaid urging me to see his Chinese reflexologist, I finally listened. I remember the first time I met Dr. Tay. He wore a white lab coat and face mask, and he seemed so serious. My reflexology session was excruciatingly painful. Every point on my feet was highly sensitive.

The kicker was when Dr. Tay told me that my reproductive system was precancerous, and he urged me to go see a gynecologist. After my session, I cried. I didn't want to go back, but I had made a deal with my husband to see Dr. Tay for one month.

Over the weeks of treatment, my body stabilized and I started to get better. Dr. Tay kept telling me to see a gynecologist, but I waved it off, thinking that I'd already been treated for the Bartholin's gland cyst, so why bother?

After a month of reflexology, I finally went to see a gynecologist. She told me there was no trace of the Bartholin's gland cyst— that there was no scarring and I had "perfect symmetry." While she was incredulous at the idea that someone could tell me that my reproductive system was precancerous simply from feeling my feet, she did say that whoever treated me did a good job.

When I reported to Dr. Tay that the gynecologist hadn't found anything wrong, he smiled and said, "Of course they didn't find anything. You've been getting reflexology."

Having experienced such an amazing recovery, I was inspired to learn the complete system of Chinese reflexology so that I could practice on myself regularly. Within a year and a half of being so sick that I wondered if I was dying, I had restored my health and was training for my first ever triathlon.

With the wisdom I have now, I know weird things like Bartholin's gland cysts don't happen if your body, mind, and spirit are in harmony. It was because I had kept putting off following my passion and holding back on expressing my brilliance that the qi in my reproductive system was blocked. In Chinese Medicine, a cyst is caused by a stagnation in the flow of qi and blood through an area, resulting in the accumulation of fluid—or in other words, the formation of a cyst.

The more I listen to my heart, follow my passion, and live my purpose, the better I feel and the more energy I have. I want you to experience amazing health and vitality too, which is why I'm so passionate about teaching you how to heal with Chinese reflexology and the mind-body connection. Together, they transformed my health and my outlook on life. I wake up every day with boundless energy and excitement, except when the cat or my kid wakes me up at 3 A.M.!

Expressing your feelings and sharing your ideas are the first steps, so let's begin with the throat point.

Chinese Reflexology Point for the Throat

Your throat is more than just a home for your voice box and a conduit for food and air. It is also the gatekeeper for expressing your emotions, voicing your thoughts, and sharing your brilliance with the world. When you hold back from expressing yourself, you block the flow of qi through your neck and throat.

In the Dragon Spirit work I do with clients, I connect with their soul energy. Because of this intense energetic connection, I often feel a physical sensation in my body when my clients are facing a deeply buried emotion.

For example, fear feels like a wave of goose bumps washing over me. Another common sensation I experience is tightness and constriction in my throat. The sensation comes about quite suddenly, and it always happens just as my client is about to express a life-changing truth, or when a repressed emotion is finally coming to the surface.

Such was the case for Julie. She was a competitive athlete. She was strong and tough, and pushed herself to excel. Years of putting on her game face had made it very difficult for her to express emotions. She didn't want to look weak. However, just because everything looked calm on the surface, it didn't mean that everything was okay on the inside.

During one of Julie's sessions, we explored a past relationship that she had long forgotten, or so she had thought. As soon as she mentioned her ex-partner, I felt a huge lump in my throat and the sensation of my throat being squeezed. Julie could barely speak. She had held back expressing so many emotions for so long that she was energetically choking herself.

As we worked together to clear these emotions and energy blocks over the course of a few weeks, I noticed a change in Julie. When I first met her, she kept her emotions tightly under wraps. However, as she became more free in expressing herself, her personality and cheekiness came bubbling up.

When you hold back your words and feelings, it creates a traffic jam of energy in your throat. And if you don't clear the energy, it can show up in your physical body as a sore throat or losing the ability to speak.

I understand this feeling intimately because I used to do this. I wouldn't allow myself to say what I felt and I certainly wouldn't let the world know how brilliant I was. People always told me, "You're so quiet." In my head, I'd be thinking, "You're so rude to say that to me," but I would never voice it aloud. Knowing what it's like to keep everything inside, I have to say that it feels so much better to speak up.

Even though voicing your emotions can make you feel vulnerable, when you do, you're actually welcoming open, honest, and authentic relationships in your life—you attract people who support you as opposed to tear you down.

You don't have to do a 180 overnight. You can start small. For example, if you don't normally speak to the cashier at the grocery store, share something about your day or what you admire about them. Or if you find yourself holding back an opinion because you don't want to make waves, go ahead and make a little splash. Your throat will thank you for it.

Singing in the shower is good, too! That's how I got my kara-oke chops. The Chinese reflexology point for the throat is also an amazing point for helping the qi to flow smoothly through your throat and neck.

What Your Throat Does

Your throat is a passageway for air and food—or depending on how you look at it, a gatekeeper to expressing your thoughts and feelings. It houses your pharynx and larynx. The pharynx is a funnel-shaped passageway connecting your nasal cavity and mouth to your esophagus (the tube where food passes to your stomach) and larynx (voice box).

Okay, I have to ask, does anyone else aside from me think that pharynx and larynx sound like made-up words from a Dr. Seuss book?

"Do you feel

the air pass through?"

asked the larynx

of the pharynx.

"I do. I do

feel the air pass through,"

said the pharynx

to the larynx.

How to Locate Your Throat Point

The reflexology point for the throat is a small circle located on the top of the foot. You'll find it in the webbing between your big toe and second toe, right at the base of the toes. The right foot corresponds with the left side of your throat, and the left foot corresponds with the right side because, as you learned in Chapter 9, your energy meridians cross over at the neck and switch sides. Interestingly, the location of this reflexology point is very similar to the acupuncture point *Liver 2*, which is used to treat sore throats.

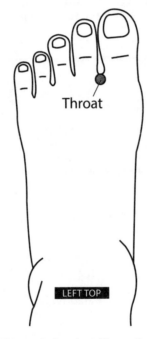

Chinese Reflexology Throat Point

How to Massage Your Throat Point

Use the knuckle of your index finger to massage the throat reflexology point. Wrap your opposite fingers under your foot to support the toes. When massaging the left foot, use your right hand for support, and your left index finger knuckle to press and twist into the point. The movement is similar to jiggling a doorknob.

When massaging the point on your right foot, switch hands— use the right knuckle to massage and the left hand for support. Massage your throat point for 15 seconds per foot.

For stronger stimulation, you can use your supporting hand to gently hold the two toes together while you press and twist. If you tend to hold back on expressing your emotions, your throat point is going to be sensitive. This point also becomes extremely sensitive when you have a sore throat, but returns to normal when your sore throat clears.

Chinese Reflexology Point for the Ovaries and Testicles

In this section, we will cover the reflexology points for both the ovaries and the testicles—the location for these points is the same. Obviously, the testicle point applies to men, and the ovary point is for women.

I find that these points tend to be some of the most sensitive points on people. I believe it's because there is a triple whammy going on for points related to the reproductive system. Whammy number one is all those mixed messages we receive about sex and our bodies. Throw in a few bad relationships and a good dose of guilt, shame, and inadequacy surrounding sex, and guess what? The result is some serious energetic blockage in the sexual organs.

Whammy number two is repression when it comes to gender roles in our society. Men are discouraged from embracing their feminine side, and women are encouraged to behave in a mas-culine way in order to succeed in the corporate world. What this ends up creating is an imbalance in the most fundamental of energies—yin and yang, the feminine and masculine.

Finally, the third whammy is that the reproductive system represents the energy of creation. This encompasses your ideas, your passions, and your soul's calling. When you hold back on expressing your brilliance, you disrupt the smooth flow of qi in your body. Stifling your ideas and creativity results in energy blocks in the ovaries, uterus, testicles, and prostate. It's a literal manifestation of holding back on your creative energies.

What the Ovaries Do

The ovaries are two small glands located on either side of the uterus. They produce and store eggs. During ovulation, a mature egg is released into a connecting fallopian tube. In addition to being part of the reproductive system, the ovaries are also part of the endocrine system. They produce estrogen and progesterone, which are hormones that help regulate menstruation and pregnancy.

What the Testicles Do

The testicles are a pair of glands located in the scrotum. Like the ovaries, they're part of both the endocrine and reproductive systems. The testicles produce the hormone testosterone, and they also produce sperm.

How to Locate Your Ovary or Testicle Point

IMPORTANT

If you are currently menstruating, do not massage this point until after your period has passed.

The location of this reflexology point is the same for both men and women. If you're a woman, this point will be for your ovaries, and if you're a man, the point will be for your testicles.

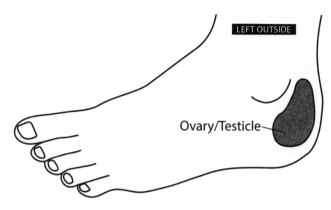

Chinese Reflexology Ovary/Testicle Point

The ovary/testicle point is a teardrop-shaped area on the outside edge of the foot. It is located just below and behind the anklebone. The right foot is for the right ovary or testicle, and the left foot is for the left ovary or testicle.

How to Massage Your Ovary or Testicle Point

Since the point is located on the outside edge of the foot, you may feel a bit awkward when you first start massaging this point. It is easier to reach the points on the outer edge when you stand up and place your foot flat on a stool or chair like you did for the knee reflexology point.

Beginning with your left foot, reach down with your left arm and use the knuckle of your index finger to press into the reflexology area for this point. Massage in an up and down motion, where up is toward your anklebone and down is toward the sole of your foot.

The skin on the side of the foot is more delicate than on the sole, so apply a thin layer of lubricant such as oil or lotion to reduce friction while massaging. Massage for a total of 15 seconds per foot.

Because there are nerves running through this area of your foot, you may experience an electric-shock sensation if you accidentally hit a nerve. The feeling will be mild and last for less than a second. After the shock has passed, use a lighter pressure to massage this point.

Chinese Reflexology Point for the Uterus and Prostate

The reflexology points for the uterus and prostate are similar to the points for the ovaries and testicles. They're located in the same position on the foot, but on the inner edge as opposed to the outer edge.

In Chinese Medicine, even though the uterus is not one of the twelve primary energy meridians, it does deserve special mention. Menstrual cramps are attributed to a stagnation in the flow of qi or blood through the uterus. In addition, consuming foods and drinks that are cold in temperature can cause cramps because the digestive tract is in close proximity to the uterus. The cold temperature can transfer to the uterus and upset the balance in this organ. So if you get menstrual cramps, don't reach for mint chocolate chip ice cream!

There isn't a similar classical TCM perspective for the prostate, but I would advise not reaching for ice cream if your friend or partner can't have any. Okay, all joking aside (I could seriously go for some organic ice cream right now), let's explore more about these two organs.

What the Uterus Does

The uterus is a hollow organ that is shaped like an upside-down pear. If you've read any books about pregnancy, you know that they love comparing the developing fetus to fruit. *Your baby is now the size of a mango.*

Pre-baby, the uterus is about the size of a pear. Once it becomes a home for a wee one, the uterus expands to accommodate the baby's growth until you feel like your uterus is the size of a water-melon. During childbirth, muscles in the uterus contract to help push the baby out of the womb and into the world. Hello, baby.

What the Prostate Does

The prostate is a walnut-sized gland located below the bladder. It produces prostatic fluid, a milky substance that is a major component of semen. While the female reproductive system is a cornucopia of fruit analogies, for some reason, the male reproductive system is often compared to assorted nuts. Maybe it's because fruits and nuts go well together.

How to Locate Your Uterus or Prostate Point

IMPORTANT

If you are currently menstruating, do not massage this point until after your period has passed.

The uterus/prostate point is very similar to the ovary/testicle point. It is also a teardrop-shaped area just below and behind the anklebone. However, instead of being on the outside edge of the foot, the uterus/prostate point is located on the inside edge.

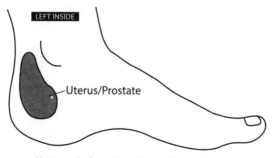

Chinese Reflexology Uterus/Prostate Point

203

How to Massage Your Uterus or Prostate Point

This point is much easier to massage than the ovary/testicle point. Because it is on the inner edge of the foot, you can sit down with your foot in your lap. Beginning with your left foot, press the knuckle of your right index finger into the reflexology area. Then massage up and down, where up is toward the anklebone and down is toward the sole of your foot. It is very common for this reflexology point to be sensitive when you massage it.

Due to the skin on the side of the foot being more delicate than the sole, and because you're using your knuckle, be sure to apply a thin layer of lubricant such as oil or lotion to reduce friction. Massage for a total of 15 seconds per foot.

Similar to the ovary/testicle point, you may feel a weird sensation if you accidentally hit a nerve while massaging this area. If that's the case, use a little bit less pressure when you massage this point.

Points to Remember

After practicing the points in this chapter, you may find yourself wanting to express your voice, opinions, and creativity more—so do it! This is so good for your qi because expressing your brilliance helps clear energetic blocks in your throat and reproductive system. Here's a quick summary of the reflexology points covered in this chapter.

1. Throat Point

- **Benefits:** clears stuck energy in the throat to alleviate a sore throat and helps with expressing thoughts and feelings
- **Location:** on the tops of both feet, in the webbing between the first two toes
- **Massage Technique:** press and twist with knuckle
- **Recommended Time:** 15 seconds per foot

2. Ovary and Testicle Point

- **Benefits:** harmonizes qi in reproductive system and helps clear creative blocks
- **Location:** teardrop-shaped area on the outside edge of both feet, below and behind the anklebone
- **Massage Technique:** apply lubricant and massage up and down (anklebone to bottom of foot direction) with knuckle
- **Recommended Time:** 15 seconds per foot

3. Uterus and Prostate Point

- **Benefits:** harmonizes qi in reproductive system and helps clear creative blocks
- **Location:** teardrop-shaped area on the inside edge of both feet, below and behind the anklebone
- **Massage Technique:** apply lubricant and massage up and down (anklebone to bottom of foot direction) with knuckle
- **Recommended Time:** 15 seconds per foot

CHAPTER 15

PUTTING IT ALL TOGETHER

Congratulations!

You now know close to two dozen reflexology points. That's almost half of the points in this system of traditional Chinese reflexology. Give yourself a pat on the back. You deserve it. Way to go! High fives! Yay!

So now that you've mastered all of these points—or are on your way to mastering them—you might be curious as to how you can apply your newly acquired knowledge to improve your health and well-being. You probably want to know how Chinese reflexology can make a difference in your day-to-day life.

These are ponderings any clever mind would want addressed—my mind sure would want to know. So let's look at this right now. Think of this chapter as the FAQ section of a website where we'll look at some of the most common questions about practicing Chinese reflexology.

Recommended Order for Massaging the Points

Let's start first by reviewing what you've learned so far. As you look over the following groups of points, try picturing in your mind where the points are located on your feet.

- **Clearing and recharging:** Kidney, Bladder, lymphatic drainage

- **Harmonizing the heart and mind:** Heart, brain, temporal area

- **Nourishing your body:** solar plexus, Spleen, Stomach

- **Restoring balance:** Liver, adrenal gland, pituitary gland

- **Embracing change:** Large Intestine (hand), rectum/ anus (hand), Lung, Gall Bladder

- **Moving forward fully supported:** shoulder, knee, inner hip, outer hip

- **Expressing your brilliance:** throat, ovary/testicle, uterus/prostate

That's 21 foot points in total (plus two hand points). If you were to regularly massage these points in the above order, you'd be all over the place, or perhaps a more apt description is that you would be all over your feet. While it is better to learn reflexology points when they are grouped by a common purpose, it's much simpler to practice the points when they are grouped by their location on your feet.

So let's revisit these points, only this time we will reorganize them and give them a *new order*—one of my favorite bands from the '80s!

Here are a few guidelines for the order in which to massage the points:

1. Massage your left foot first and then do your right foot.

2. Begin with the points in the excretory system. Always start with the Kidney first.

3. For the remaining points, I find it convenient to massage all of the points on one side of the foot before moving on to the next side. Here is the order that I recommend:

   - Points on inner edge of foot

   - Points on sole of foot

   - Points on outer edge of foot

   - Points on top of foot

   - Hand points (optional)

Now I'm going to toss in one more variable. Since you're practicing the gentle method of Chinese reflexology, it's a lot to massage over 20 points in one sitting. If you practiced them all at once, your fingers, knuckles, and thumbs would get tired very quickly. This might actually discourage you from practicing regularly, and we don't want that to happen.

With a reflexology stick, it would be easy to massage all of the points without getting tired because the stick gives you leverage to press harder, and thus reduce the time and effort required to massage your points.

However, there is a way to make the gentle method easier. I created two core routines that you can practice using the gentle method. Each routine contains about a dozen reflexology foot points, which is a very manageable number of points to massage in one session.

Core Routine #1: Points to Massage

1. Kidney
2. Bladder
3. Brain
4. Temporal area
5. Lung
6. Shoulder
7. Solar plexus
8. Stomach
9. Heart (left foot only)
10. Spleen (left foot only)
11. Throat
12. Lymphatic drainage

Core Routine #2: Points to Massage

1. Kidney
2. Adrenal gland
3. Bladder
4. Inner hip
5. Uterus/prostate
6. Pituitary gland
7. Liver (right foot only)
8. Gall Bladder (right foot only)
9. Knee
10. Outer hip
11. Ovary/testicle
12. Optional hand points (Large Intestine, rectum/anus)

Ideally, you would alternate routines every other day. This would be equivalent to practicing all of the points that you've learned twice a week. Here's a sample week:

- Sunday: Routine #1
- Monday: Rest
- Tuesday: Routine #2
- Wednesday: Rest
- Thursday: Routine #1
- Friday: Rest
- Saturday: Routine #2

When you reach the end of the week, you can choose to make the following Sunday a rest day so that you can continue practicing every other day. Alternately, you can repeat the routine outlined above and practice Routine #1 on the Sunday.

If your life is super busy or if you're a little lazy (it's okay—be honest!), instead of practicing every other day, you could choose to practice each routine only once a week. Here's a sample week:

- Sunday: Routine #1
- Monday: Rest
- Tuesday: Chill out
- Wednesday: Routine #2
- Thursday: Do nothing
- Friday: Relax
- Saturday: Party!

I'll leave the choice up to you, and hopefully your Gall Bladder qi will help you make the decision. Your body will return to balance faster when you massage your feet every other day as opposed to only twice a week. However, if you can't make the commitment at this time, as I always tell my students, "Some reflexology is better than no reflexology."

If you find that even a dozen points is too much to manage at this time, then at the very least, massage the points for the energy meridians of the body (Kidney, Bladder, Lung, Stomach, Heart, and Spleen in Routine 1; and Kidney, Bladder, Liver, and Gall Bladder in Routine 2). In addition, massage the brain and lymphatic drainage points.

For your convenience, you'll find a Quick Reference Table, containing all of the foot points you've learned, in the Resources section at the end of this book. The table lists the points in the order in which to massage them, along with their corresponding location, massage technique, and recommended massage times.

Tracking Your Progress

It wouldn't be any fun for your mind if there wasn't some way to measure your progress. My mind loves sticker charts and admittedly so does my heart. It appeals to the little kid in me. So I created a Track Your Progress chart for you to keep track of improvements in your qi.

Take a moment now to fill out the chart. Write down today's date and then rate all of your reflexology points on a scale from 0 to 10. This is a rating system similar to the one you used in Chapter 2, only this scale goes up to ten to allow for more precision in your ratings. A rating of zero would mean that you don't feel any sensitivity. One would be for a slightly uncomfortable point. Ten is for a @#%! point that feels extremely painful even with light pressure.

I personally prefer not writing in books, but that certainly hasn't stopped me from folding corners on pages. If you'd rather not write on the page, or if you're reading a digital version of this book, you can quickly jot down your points and ratings on a sheet of paper. Go ahead and do it now. You'll need your ratings in just a short while.

You can also download a copy of the Track Your Progress chart from my website at www.chinesefootreflexology.com/track yourprogress.

Track Your Progress Chart

TRACK YOUR PROGRESS	Date:		Date:	
Reflexology Points for Routine #1	Left Foot	Right Foot	Left Foot	Right Foot
Kidney (Chapter 8)				
Bladder (Chapter 8)				
Brain (Chapter 9)				
Temporal Area (Chapter 9)				
Lung (Chapter 12)				
Shoulder (Chapter 13)				
Solar Plexus (Chapter 10)				
Stomach (Chapter 10)				
Heart (Chapter 9)		▓		▓
Spleen (Chapter 10)		▓		▓
Throat (Chapter 14)				
Lymphatic Drainage (Chapter 8)				
Place Star Here				

TRACK YOUR PROGRESS	Date:		Date:	
Reflexology Points for Routine #2	Left Foot	Right Foot	Left Foot	Right Foot
Kidney (Chapter 8)				
Adrenal Gland (Chapter 11)				
Bladder (Chapter 8)				
Inner Hip (Chapter 13)				
Uterus/Prostate (Chapter 14)				
Pituitary Gland (Chapter 11)				
Liver (Chapter 11)	■		■	
Gall Bladder (Chapter 12)	■		■	
Knee (Chapter 13)				
Outer Hip (Chapter 13)				
Ovary/Testicle (Chapter 14)				
Place Star Here				

Note: The hand points are not included in this chart because it is difficult to accurately gauge the sensitivity of points on your hands.

After rating your points, revisit this chart in about six to eight weeks and rate your points again. As long as you massage all of your points regularly, abstain from drinking alcohol, get enough rest, and eat a reasonably healthy diet, you should see a reduction in the sensitivity of your points. This indicates an improvement in the flow of qi. In a two-month time frame practicing the gentle method, a rating reduction of 1 or 2 is really good, and 3 or 4 is amazing.

Initially, you want to aim for a point sensitivity level in the range of 3 or less. When *all of your points* reach this level, you can reduce the number of times you practice the Chinese reflexology core routines. But you can also continue your regular practice if you prefer.

Practicing both routines twice a month is good for maintenance. Even though I massage all of my reflexology points a couple times a month, I find that I'm usually rubbing my feet daily depending on what curveballs are thrown my way. For example, if my son catches a cold at school, I'll rub my Lung point to boost my defensive qi so that I don't catch his cold. Rubbing my feet has become a way of life for me and my family—and I often hear this from my students, too.

Ideally, you want your points to rate at a zero because this would indicate a total balance of qi in your body. But if you were in this state, you wouldn't care what your ratings were!

One other thing to mention is that your mind may be overly critical if you don't see amazing progress for all of your points. However, your body simply does not heal this way. Some points may improve faster than others. And if you've recently been under stress or haven't had enough sleep, some points may be temporarily worse.

What matters most is that you see an overall trend of improvement. This tracking chart can also help motivate you to practice regularly. Be sure to give yourself a star for an A+ effort when you've finished rating your points.

Chinese Reflexology Foot Charts

You may be wondering, since you've learned close to half of the points in this system of Chinese reflexology, what about the other points? Which points haven't you learned yet, and where are they located?

First, I'd like to remind you that I chose the points in this book because they are some of the most powerful all-purpose reflexology points, and also the easiest ones to learn without actually observing how to massage them in an online video or in person. These points give you a lot of proverbial bang for your buck, or return for your effort.

To satisfy your curiosity about the other points, you'll find complete Chinese reflexology foot charts in the Resources section. Theses charts will show you the locations for all of the reflexology points in this system. However, please only practice the points that you've learned so far.

Which Points Should You Massage for a Specific Health Concern?

People often tell me about their health issues and then ask which points they should massage. They'll ask me this even if they've already received a series of free e-mail lessons from my website, yet they haven't started massaging their feet regularly. Grasshopper, first you must walk; then you can run.

The points you've learned so far are some of the most powerful points for improving your overall health and vitality. Start with these first. Get into a regular routine to strengthen your body's qi. Regardless of whether you have early stage macular degeneration or a bladder infection, the foundation for true healing is built upon improving your overall health. The true essence of Chinese reflexology isn't about picking points for a specific disease. It's about healing and balancing as a whole.

In an ideal world, I would recommend that you learn and practice all of the points in this system of traditional Chinese reflexology. The whole is greater than the sum of its parts. However, with what you've learned so far, you have enough points to make a big difference in improving the flow of qi in your body. So practice regularly and when you're ready to run, there's always the Chinese Reflexology Sole Mastery Program.

But there is something else you can do to power up what you've learned . . .

Increasing Massage Times for Specific Points

In addition to practicing the recommended reflexology routines, you can add extra massage time for the points that your body needs the most. However, you have to proceed slowly, as there are some points that can trigger detox symptoms if you massage them too much.

For long-standing issues, it really is most beneficial to practice the complete system of Chinese reflexology with a reflexology stick. However, your body can let you know if there are points that would benefit from additional massage time. But before you add extra time, you must be ready. If you can answer *yes* to both of the following questions, then you're ready to add extra time.

1. Are you practicing regularly?

You can answer *yes* to this question if you've been practicing the two reflexology routines every other day for at least six weeks. It's okay if you missed one or two sessions during the six-week period. However, if you missed three or more sessions, keep practicing until you reach six weeks without missing more than two sessions in total.

You can also answer *yes* if you have been practicing both routines at least once a week for eight consecutive weeks, and have not missed more than two sessions during this period of time. If you have been unable to practice this often, then you're not ready to add extra massage time.

2. Are you free from detox symptoms or other side effects?

As you've been regularly massaging your feet, have you been free from detox symptoms such as headaches, fatigue, fever, irritability, rash, or other skin breakouts? Have you also been free from other side effects such as achy feet, skin irritation, bruises, emotional reactions, or minor short-term aches in your body?

If you've generally felt fine after practicing reflexology, then you can answer *yes* to this question. If you're not sure, then skip the additional massage time for now.

How to Identify Points That Would Benefit from Extra Massage

If you're wondering which reflexology points should get extra attention, this is a question that is not up to me to answer. It's up to your feet. Remember way back in Chapter 2 when I told you that your feet are a source of wisdom? Your feet will tell you which are the most beneficial reflexology points for you to massage based on the sensitivity of your points. So take a look at your Track Your Progress chart. (Oops, did you not complete it yet? That's okay. Go ahead and do it now.)

Looking at your chart, identify your top five most sensitive points. These are the points that you should massage. If you have more than five highly sensitive points, choose the points that correspond to the primary energy meridians in Chinese Medicine. If there are more than five of these, then pick the points highest up on the following list:

1. Kidney
2. Bladder
3. Spleen
4. Liver
5. Lung

6. Stomach

7. Heart

8. Gall Bladder

As points become less sensitive, you can stop adding extra time for them and move on to the other points that feel more sensitive. This way you'll always have a rotation of five points that get extra massage time. I would not recommend adding additional time for more than five points, as this would increase the likelihood of triggering detox symptoms or side effects, as discussed in Chapter 7. You can, however, choose fewer than five points for adding extra massage time—you could even pick just one or two.

How Much Extra Time Should You Add?

For each of your top five (or fewer) points, add 15 seconds per point during your regular reflexology routine. If you feel fine afterward (for the rest of the day and the next day) and do not experience any detox symptoms or side effects, then you can add an additional 15 seconds the next time you massage these points as part of your routine.

Continue adding time in increments of 15 seconds until you feel you've had enough (listen to your body instead of your brain) or you reach a *maximum of three minutes per point in one day*, whichever comes first. Now, just because I wrote *three minutes* here, don't take that as free license to jump in and massage a point for this amount of time right away. I appreciate your enthusiasm, but you have to gradually build up to this length of time, and you should only massage this long for a maximum of five different reflexology points.

As you gradually increase the massage time, you will also be building up strength and endurance in your hands to massage your points. If, however, at any time your fingers, thumbs, or knuckles feel tired, please rest your hands and only massage for the amount of time that feels comfortable.

Another thing to note is that when you are massaging a point for over 60 seconds (even the ones on the soles of your feet), it's a good idea to apply a lubricant such as massage oil. This will help minimize friction and reduce the chance of irritating your skin.

You can also increase the stimulation of a reflexology point by gradually increasing the amount of pressure you apply when massaging the point—just like you would for adding extra time. Press a little bit harder, and if you don't experience any detox symptoms or side effects (or tired fingers, thumbs, or knuckles), then you can use a little more pressure the next time you massage. Stronger and more intense pressure helps you progress faster over a shorter period of time. That's what makes a reflexology stick so powerfully efficient.

While it may be tempting to go full force right away, a balanced and gentle approach will benefit your health the most over the long run. When you overdo it, you increase the likelihood of triggering detox symptoms or side effects—and you also risk burning out, which could cause you to stop practicing reflexology altogether.

Think of it like paddling a canoe toward an island in the center of a large lake. Sure, you could start off paddling as hard as you can, but at some point, you're going to get tired and need a rest. Then you'll take your paddle out of the water and float around aimlessly. You might completely drift off course and end up having to paddle even harder to reach your destination.

On the other hand, if you guide your canoe with a slow and steady pace, you can keep paddling for however long it takes to reach your destination. In the meantime, you'll be relaxed and enjoying the scenery for the entire trip.

Chinese Reflexology Mini Routines

The gradual increase in massage time and pressure applies primarily to your practice of the two core routines. There are times, however, when you can massage a select number of points for longer than what is specified in the core routines. This applies to short-term health issues that are usually mild and temporary in nature.

In the Resources section at the end of this book, you'll find a variety of mini reflexology routines for these types of health issues, such as the common cold, indigestion, insomnia, and stress. Mini routines contain a small subset of the points you've learned so far. You can practice these mini routines in addition to the core reflexology routines unless otherwise noted.

Is It Possible to Overstimulate a Point?

Absolutely! When you massage your reflexology points too much, you increase the risk of experiencing detox symptoms. Don't overdo it. Instead, follow the guidelines in this book for practicing the core routines and mini reflexology routines. Chinese reflexology works best when you practice regularly over time. It is better to massage your feet for ten minutes, six weeks in a row, rather than 60 minutes all at once.

Health and vitality are about achieving balance in your body. Healing is as much about the mental and emotional aspects as it is about the physical. You cannot restore harmony if you act in ways that are not harmonious.

Excessively massaging your reflexology points is an act based in fear, and it indicates a lack of faith in your body's natural healing process. You're afraid that you won't get better right away, so you feel compelled to massage your points too much.

Let go of the fear—take a deep breath and release it now.

When Will You Notice a Difference?

In the very moment that you begin rubbing your feet, things start shifting at the energy level. The effects are subtle, and you may not notice them right away, especially if you've been feeling disconnected from your body lately. You can, however, observe the effects if you know where to look and what you're looking for.

One of the easiest ways for you to recognize the effects of reflexology is to compare your feet before and after you massage them. Massage your left foot first, and then compare it to your right foot *before* you massage it.

Compare the feet by pressing the soles together. You'll notice that your left foot will feel much warmer than the right. In addition, when you compare the color of one foot to the other, you will see that the foot you massaged looks rosier, whereas the other may look and feel like a cold fish!

These signs indicate an increase in the flow of qi and blood through the foot that you massaged, as well as the corresponding body parts and energy meridians. If you are someone who is very aware of your energy, you may also notice a sense of lightness in your body, a tingly feeling all over, or the sensation that your cells are buzzing with energy.

What You'll Notice in Three to Four Weeks

If you have been practicing regularly every other day, you'll notice in about three to four weeks that your reflexology points feel less sensitive when you press on them. Of course, you'll have to be eating reasonably well and getting enough rest, too.

At first, you may wonder if you are simply getting used to the discomfort because you've been massaging your feet so much. Let me assure you that this is not the case. Your reflexology points would feel exactly the same if there were no changes happening with the flow of energy in your body. So you are definitely not imagining it when your points feel less sensitive. The reduction in sensitivity indicates that you are getting stronger and healthier at the energy level. And when your energy is flowing as it should, your physical health will follow.

What You'll Notice in Six to Eight Weeks

As you continue to massage your feet regularly, the reduction in the sensitivity of your reflexology points will become even more pronounced. It will reach a level that you can measure and take note of in your Track Your Progress chart. While you may give some points the same rating as before, others may show significant improvement, but don't expect the numbers to go from an 8 down to a 3 in just a few weeks. A reduction of 1 to 2 points is actually a huge improvement!

When you can gauge a reduction in the sensitivity of your points even if it is a "tiny" one, this is a sign that changes are happening at the physical level. As the qi improves, your physical body improves. Long-term conditions with their roots in energy imbalances will start to shift (*hint:* almost everything has its roots in an energy imbalance).

At this stage, you should begin seeing subtle changes at the physical level. How this manifests is different for everyone, and it may not be in the shape or form that you expect because expectations come from your mind, not your body.

Some people will feel an overall improvement in their health—they'll sleep better and feel calmer and more energized. Others may notice changes in their digestion, such as less bloating when they eat, a moderation of food cravings, or more regularity with their bowel movements.

And others may not notice anything at all. It is the *absence of symptoms* that often takes longer for someone to notice. Such was the case for me when I began practicing reflexology. It took me two years before I realized that I no longer experienced neck and shoulder pain from my car accident.

Rest assured, if your reflexology points are feeling less sensitive, then healing is happening in your body. Your mind just doesn't have any control over it. But your body knows what it's doing, and it is healing at exactly the pace and order in which it needs to.

What If Your Sensitivity Ratings Don't Go Down?

Very rarely, I come across people who massage their feet regularly but don't see a reduction in the sensitivity levels of their reflexology points. It is usually because they are still doing something that is at the energetic root of the qi imbalance in their body. For example, if you're allergic to shellfish, but you insist on eating it, then you're not giving your body space to heal.

Holding on to emotional pain can also counteract the effects of reflexology. No matter how much you massage your feet, the qi disharmony will still be there until you address the emotions. For example, if you are nearsighted, your vision cannot dramatically improve (without corrective lenses or surgery) until you make peace with the emotions that preceded the blurring of your vision.

There may also be something in your lifestyle that aggravates your health. I remember two clients who showed very little improvement. One was a smoker, and the other binge drank on the weekends and spent way too much time working. Neither was willing to change their habits despite my encouragement, and this was reflected by the sensitivity levels of the points in their feet.

Reflexology points may also remain sensitive if your body needs more time to heal (see the section below). Chronic issues often take longer to heal, and you may need a kick start to get back into balance. If that's the case, then please see your physician or health practitioner.

Even if you do not see a reduction in the sensitivity of your points, Chinese reflexology is still beneficial to practice. Remember the analogy I gave you of scooping water out of a leaky boat? When you massage the points on your feet, it helps keep your boat afloat, giving you time to figure out how to *repair* the boat. And that's why I recommend that you continue massaging your points but also visit your physician or health practitioner to see if they may have the materials that you need to fix your boat.

Other Factors That Influence Healing

While Chinese reflexology supports healing at the energy level, there are other factors that also influence the body's healing process.

- **Overall health and resilience:** The stronger, healthier, and more resilient you are, the quicker you heal.

- **Age:** Generally speaking, younger people heal faster than older people.

- **Chronic vs. acute conditions:** The less time you have had a condition, the easier it is to release it. Some conditions may seem like they're acute because they come on quite suddenly, but they are actually chronic because they have their roots in long-term energy imbalances. My Bartholin's gland cyst is a good example. It happened suddenly and was resolved in just a few weeks. However, I would classify it as chronic because the cyst was a result of qi disharmonies that had been going on for years.

- **Diet and nutrition:** Eating and drinking foods that support your body, and avoiding those that are harmful (e.g., alcohol), helps you to heal faster.

- **Stress levels and lifestyle:** Chronic stress and not getting enough rest deplete your body's resilience and thus make it harder for your body to bounce back. Living a balanced life contributes to your body's overall health and resilience.

- **Underlying mental and emotional roots:** If your mind keeps replaying the negative emotions or backstory behind a condition, then it is difficult for your body to release the physical manifestation of your thoughts. However, if you are willing to shift

your thinking and release old emotional wounds,
then it is easier for your body to return to balance.

- **Congenital jing:** If you inherited a hearty amount of life force energy from your parents (they were strong and healthy and made a substantial deposit into your energy trust fund when you were born), then your body can draw upon this reserve to heal itself.

Regardless of the current state of your body, life, or health, Chinese reflexology is the cornerstone for healing with energy. Practice consistently over time to create a solid and strong foundation for lifelong health and vitality. While a journey of a thousand miles begins with a single step, you make extraordinary progress on that journey when you keep moving forward—and by this section of the book, you're well on your way. Kudos to you!

Now it's time to take a giant step forward with the third catalyst—following your heart and soul. It's the most powerful catalyst of them all. So take a deep breath, and when you're ready, turn the page. In the next section, I'll show you how to connect with your Dragon Spirit to balance your body, mind, heart, and spirit.

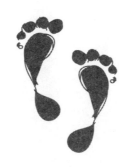

THE THIRD CATALYST

FOLLOWING YOUR
HEART AND SOUL

CHAPTER 16

How to Connect with Your Dragon Spirit

So I've shared quite a few stories in this book about how connecting with my Dragon Spirit transformed my health and that of my clients. When I started listening to my inner wisdom, that's when the magic happened. Healing became effortless because this connection with my Dragon Spirit is my direct line for receiving the rejuvenating energy of the Universe.

My Dragon Spirit also led me to hear my heart's calling, and it gave me guidance so that my soul path manifested easily and effortlessly—as compared with when I tried to make it happen with my mind. The more I follow my passions, the more energy I have and the healthier I feel. And that, my friends, is how the third catalyst, following your heart and soul, is the most powerful catalyst of them all for health and vitality—it enables you to *thrive*.

Everyone has a Dragon Spirit inside them—*even you*. How would *you* like to connect with *your* Dragon Spirit?

When you hear the voice of your Dragon Spirit, it gives you clarity. It lets you know what is helping your body and what is harming your body. You feel more in tune with your physical self, so that you are much more likely to get enough sleep, eat nourishing foods, and feel motivated to exercise—all wonderful things for boosting your qi and helping it flow smoothly through your energy meridians.

You'll also feel more grounded, both mentally and emotionally. This will make you less likely to put yourself in stressful situations, and more likely to seek balance in your life. And as you feel more balance, your energy vibration rises, and it becomes easier to see the most expansive path for you to follow your bliss—leading to a very positive self-perpetuating energy cycle.

Fine-tuning Your Connection

If you're not used to listening to your inner wisdom, you might not know whether the voice you hear is your intuition speaking or your mind. You may even wonder if the Universe and all that talk of interconnectedness, oneness, and manifesting your reality is really *real*.

I've met many people who were quite adamant that they didn't have an inner voice and that they never received any signs from the Universe. However, after I probed them with a few questions, they suddenly remembered a "coincidence" that happened to them or a time when they had a gut feeling about a situation that turned out to be correct.

This certainly applied to Paul. Like many of my clients, he was highly intelligent and very analytical. Instead of hearing an inner voice, Paul heard his mind going around in circles. You could say it had a mind of its own!

As a result, Paul felt completely cut off from his inner guidance. While others would see signs and messages from the Universe, his view was bleak and empty. Many of his thoughts were despondent, filled with guilt, worry, and disappointment.

When he contracted Lyme disease, it became chronic and was accompanied by excruciating pain throughout his body.

His hands were especially susceptible to the pain, and his veins became inflamed on a regular basis.

Paul lived in constant pain. When I tested his reflexology points, he reported sensitivity levels that were *lower* than I expected. He was so used to enduring intense levels of agony that he had an unusually high tolerance for pain.

When Paul first came to see me, he was monotone and listless. He was certain that the Universe had forsaken him and left him to suffer. His mind was so dominant that it stopped him from recognizing his own inner voice and guidance.

But what brought him to me, if not his heart and soul? As he spoke about feeling like he had reached the point of giving up, it was clear that he hadn't—otherwise he wouldn't have come to see me. The Universe had led him to me, and his heart had guided him to his first Chinese reflexology session.

It was a random series of "coincidences" that led him to my website. It took many more months before he contacted me to schedule an appointment. The first time, his mind ran interference and he cancelled. But a year later, he contacted me again, and this time he kept his appointment.

In addition to addressing the qi imbalances in his body, I recognized that Paul needed assistance with reining in his mind. His thoughts were fixated on his condition—and justifiably so after suffering for so many years. However, in order for his body to heal, we had to reignite the flames of hope.

Paul felt like the Universe had left him to his own devices. However, as I got to know him, he shared stories about various "coincidences" that had led him to different healing experiences. I pointed out that they were not by chance, but were actually signs that the Universe was guiding him. He seemed a little surprised to hear this, but even under logical scrutiny, there were too many coincidences, gut feelings, and happenstances to dismiss it.

Over the course of several weeks, I began to see a shift in Paul's perspective. As he got better at controlling his mind, as opposed to his mind controlling him, he started listening to his hunches and feelings more.

One day, he told me how he happened to see a flyer for a Constellation Therapy workshop. He'd seen a similar flyer a long time ago, but this time he acted on it. The workshop was fully booked, but at the last minute, there was a cancellation and a space opened up for him. After attending the workshop, he experienced another huge breakthrough in his healing.

Sometimes Paul would forget about these events and occurrences. That's one way the mind stays in charge—it conveniently forgets life-shifting moments. However, I would gently remind him whenever he expressed that the Universe wasn't there for him. Presented logically, Paul's mind couldn't argue with the many helpful occurrences in his life.

And as he began to see that he did indeed have an inner voice, and he had always had one (he had been a sensitive child), he began to see himself differently. His despondency gradually shifted to allow a forgotten feeling to blossom—hope. And with hope, he became more confident in trusting his inner guidance and listening to his feelings to determine who to see or what to do to help him recover from the chronic Lyme disease.

Instead of handing his health over to others, he began charting his own course and trusting his own guidance more. And surprise, surprise (really no surprise at all), the pain receded and Paul started to get better. His outlook brightened, and he began looking forward to the future.

Just like Paul, your life is filled with "coincidences" and moments of intuition, too. There are signs everywhere of your inner voice guiding you with support from the Universe. If you find this hard to believe, it's only because your mind has analyzed your experiences to death—quite literally—so that you discount and dismiss them. However, once you start paying attention, and maybe even writing them down so that you don't forget them, you will start to see yourself differently. Then you'll be connecting with *your* Dragon Spirit, and the more you listen, the more you'll hear it.

Your Dragon Spirit Playbook

Most people think that they can't hear their inner voice because it's not loud enough. They expect guidance from the Universe to sound like bellowing through a megaphone. If that happened all the time, it would be insanely freaky.

Hearing a loud voice usually only occurs during a time of crisis or when the Universe needs to hit you over the head because you've been a stubborn mule. Most of the time, your inner voice is as quiet as a whisper.

Even though you are always connected to the Universe, you may not feel it because of the nonstop chatter of your mind. It's like driving with a dirty windshield. The freeway and road signs are out there, but you need a clean window in order to see where you're going. The same is true for your inner guidance. It's there for you, but you need to clear some mind clutter in order to hear it.

Our minds create smoke screens because change can feel scary. Our minds want proof that change will make our lives better. It needs to have everything figured out in advance—every single step and every possible consequence, including a guaranteed outcome—before feeling at ease with embarking on a new journey.

On the other hand, your heart doesn't need this. It knows that no matter what you do or how it plays out, you will be okay. What matters more is the journey. Instead of stressing over a choice, your Dragon Spirit guides you forward. It *loves* adventure and exploration.

The best way to connect with your Dragon Spirit is to quiet your mind so that you can hear the stillness within. It is in the stillness that your intuition speaks. It is in the stillness that the qi flows. And it is in the stillness that you live and thrive.

So to help you along, I'm going to give you a Dragon Spirit playbook with six ways to quiet your mind so that you can connect with your inner wisdom. I'm also going to share these ways with you within the context of martial arts because one of your mind's best tactics for avoiding change is to conveniently "forget" what you've just read. By bringing in the martial arts connection, you'll have another way to anchor the information in your memory. No martial arts experience necessary!

Strategy #1: Know Your Opponent's Strengths and Weaknesses

Before sparring with an opponent in karate, I always took into account their belt rank and how long they had been practicing. The belt rank let me know which techniques they'd already learned and what I could expect in the fight. How long they'd been practicing let me know how *well* they knew the techniques.

So let's take an assessment of our minds. Even though I use the term *opponent,* I want to remind you that the mind is not your adversary. It's like being in karate class where sparring partners help you reach your goal of becoming a better martial artist.

Let's start with the mind's weaknesses. You already know that the mind resists change and this shows up as fear and judgment. Your mind also likes to be in control, but when it's in charge, it tends to repeat behaviors and thought patterns that may not necessarily be in your best interest.

Now let's move on to the mind's strengths. Your mind is intelligent and analytical, and it's also a hard worker. It will keep working away at a problem until it figures out the solution, or it exhausts you, whichever comes first. The downside is that this can result in you expending more effort than necessary, and thus depleting your qi.

The key to getting your mind to work *for* you is to lead with your heart, but to give your mind tasks that leverage its strengths. For example, if you wanted to switch jobs, let your heart choose your career path, but then let your mind exercise its analytical muscle by giving it the tasks of researching the industry and putting together a kick-ass résumé.

Strategy #2: Use Speed to Your Advantage

As a petite Asian woman, I would feel intimidated by sparring partners who towered over me. Taller opponents had longer limbs, which meant that they could start kicking and punching me before I could even get near them.

However, I learned that the way to get around this was to move faster than my opponent. If I jumped in fast and close, then I could be the one punching and kicking while my taller opponent's limbs were all bunched up in the closer range.

Fast moves also work well for getting ahead of your mind. After you receive direction from your heart, it is imperative that you act on it immediately. The longer you wait, the more likely your mind will come up with excuses, fears, or judgments to hold you back.

Just jump in and take action right away. While your mind is busy assessing the outcome of your action, that's when you make your next move, and you keep moving so that you are always one step ahead of your mind.

Strategy #3: Fake Out Your Opponent

One of the best sparring tactics I learned was to throw two punches in a row. The first would be a fake to the face, followed almost immediately by a blow to the body. While my opponent was preoccupied with the fist in front of his face, he inevitably missed seeing the punch to the gut (by the way, we didn't hit hard when sparring, so nobody really got hurt).

You can do the same with your mind. Give it something to deflect its attention from what you really want to do. When your mind is engrossed, it is not as focused on resisting the changes you want in your life. The mind is quiet when it is preoccupied, and this enables you to hear your inner voice more clearly. As well, when your mind is busy, it has less time to worry and fixate on potential problems.

You can distract your mind in a couple of different ways. One way is to do activities that involve thinking, such as solving puzzles (e.g., crosswords, sudoku), reading, or learning something new. The other way is to participate in activities that are so engrossing that they free you from thinking. This includes anything that requires your full attention, such as mountain biking, cooking, crafting, working with your hands, or playing an instrument. Whenever you feel worry or fear about a new direction, simply do something that actively occupies your mind.

Strategy #4: Take It Outside

In addition to learning karate, I also studied tai chi. It is considered a "soft" style of martial arts because of its flowing moves and emphasis on cultivating internal strength over building a hard body. Because of the inward focus, I had a much greater awareness of the sensations in my body as I practiced. One thing I noticed was that there was a huge difference in how I felt when we practiced outside as opposed to in a gymnasium. In the outdoors, I felt more connected, solid, and grounded. It felt more *natural.*

Immersing yourself in nature activates your senses to keep your mind engaged. The smell of the grass, the sound of birds chirping, and the feel of a breeze across your skin help to silence the mind's chatter.

Being outside also helps recalibrate your body's energetic vibration and rebalance your qi. Your body's energetic vibration is lowered by worry, stress, and poor lifestyle choices. When you are in nature, you are surrounded by the higher frequency of the great outdoors. Since this is your body's natural vibration, it wants to recalibrate to this frequency. As you raise your vibration, this brings you more in tune with the Universe; and when you're on the same wavelength, it is much easier for the Universe to communicate with you.

Strategy #5: Know When to Walk Away

One of the paradoxes of martial arts is that you're learning how to fight, but at its highest level, martial arts is really about *not* fighting. When faced with a confrontation, the best strategy is to walk away. A true martial artist would choose not to fight.

If you ever find yourself overthinking things, walk away from the situation and do something completely different. Take a break for a cup of tea. Go for a walk. Watch a comedy. Have a nap.

How many times have you struggled with a problem and then gone to sleep and woken up with the answer? That's how your intuition speaks to you. It speaks in the moments of stillness when you stop thinking so much.

Strategy #6: Practice Until It Becomes Second Nature

When I first began karate, I learned that if I was in my head too much, it was a lot harder to learn a new technique. When I *thought* too much about how to throw a punch, I was abysmal at it. However, when I practiced repeatedly, throwing punch after punch to the point of exhaustion where my mind was too tired to think, that's when the punch became second nature. Hundreds of punches made it possible for me to automatically throw one when I saw an opening in my opponent's defenses.

Hearing your inner guidance also takes practice to become second nature. You have to practice the skill of discerning your inner voice from the chatter of your mind. The mind's language includes phrases such as *I think* and *I should*. Notice when you precede a thought or sentence with these words. It's a sign that your mind is in control.

Your soul communicates in a way that transcends words. Intuition doesn't come from thinking. It comes from *feeling*. Sure, your inner voice may still use words to pass you a message, but the words will be accompanied by a resonance in your body. You'll *hear* it in your voice and *feel* it in your body.

You can speak out loud to figure out whether a thought comes from your mind or from your soul. The thought that comes from your soul has a deeper resonance in your body when spoken out loud. Your voice sounds fuller, richer, and stronger. The words feel anchored and grounded, like they're coming from the core of your body.

For example, let's say you could choose to be either a lawyer or a dancer. I know for some being a lawyer is their heart's passion, but for this example, let's say it is the mind's choice. When you talk about becoming a dancer, you'll *feel energy* in your body, hear your voice come alive, and if you look in the mirror, you'll see your eyes sparkle.

On the other hand, when you talk about becoming a lawyer, you'll notice your energy level goes way down, and you'll find yourself saying things like, "*I think* I want to be a lawyer." You will not hear conviction in your statement. Instead your voice will sound thin and weak, like it's coming from your throat and not your core.

Inner Guidance and Interconnection

Even though the voice of your inner guidance may be very subtle in nature, you'll feel it in your heart and in every cell of your body. Your inner voice is often your first thought and feeling, and it will gently persist without evoking fear or worry. That's how you know you're on the right track.

When I finished my first draft of this book, my inner voice told me to ask one of my former acupuncture professors to review the manuscript. Immediately, Dr. Ning X. Fu came to mind. Dr. Fu is a fifth generation Chinese Medicine doctor, and her father was a very famous TCM doctor in China. When I studied TCM, Dr. Fu was a senior professor and doctoral advisor for Five Branches University, one of the top TCM schools in the United States.

Despite these formidable credentials, my rational mind discarded the idea of asking her because I knew how busy she was at her clinic. I didn't want to impose upon her. So I ran through a list of other professors in my mind, but no one else *felt right.* The thought of Dr. Fu kept persisting in my mind until I finally asked my husband to mention it to her at his upcoming acupuncture appointment and gauge her reaction.

I needn't have worried about being an imposition. Dr. Fu was *thrilled* to review my manuscript. I e-mailed her a copy, and over the course of several weeks, she read through my book and also meticulously compared the locations and indications of the reflexology points to acupuncture points. Unknown to me, Dr. Fu was also conducting research on herself . . .

When I met Dr. Fu at her clinic to get her feedback, she had a sly grin on her face as she announced that she had some research to share with me. My curiosity was piqued, but I was left hanging for several minutes when she told me to wait and then disappeared behind a closed door. A few minutes later, she emerged carrying a book written in Chinese. She told me that the book's title translated as *The Clinical Application of Acupuncture Points,* and the book contained a collection of research studies on the efficacy and application of different acupuncture points.

She turned to a page that referenced a study on the acupuncture points *Liver 3* and *Liver 4.* The study found that these points helped normalize eosinophil levels in the blood. Yes, this is getting really technical, but bear with me because a geek-out moment is about to happen.

Eosinophils are a type of white blood cell. People with allergies have elevated eosinophil levels, which indicates the imbalance in their immune system. If you recall, the lymphatic system plays an important role in supporting the immune system. Now here's the geek-out moment—*Liver 3 is located on the Chinese reflexology point for lymphatic drainage.*

Dr. Fu instantly recognized the synergies between *Liver 3* and the lymphatic drainage point, so she decided to do a little research on herself. She told me she had suffered from skin allergies for many years, and whenever she had her blood tested, her absolute eosinophil count was very high. A normal count is 500 cells (or less) per milliliter (mL) of blood. Dr. Fu's blood usually tested much higher in the range of 600 to 1,000 cells/mL. After reading my book, Dr. Fu began regularly massaging the lymphatic drainage points on her feet. She told me it was too difficult to needle herself (practice self-acupuncture), because she was always on the go treating her patients. However, it was very convenient for her to massage her feet for a few seconds here and there throughout the day.

A few weeks later, she had her blood tested. When the results came in, she was delighted that her absolute eosinophil count was under 500 for the first time in years. She was even more thrilled that her allergies were much improved. Her skin was healing—it was no longer as sensitive, and her skin breakouts were clearing up, too.

She grinned broadly as she stated, "I know your book is going to help. It's been *proven* to help. I tested it on myself. Now I'm teaching my patients to do your techniques at home and practice on themselves. Acupuncture is good, but people can't needle themselves. With Chinese reflexology, you can do it anytime, anyplace. It's much easier, it's economical, and it's so convenient."

Wow! I was moved beyond words by her enthusiasm, and my heart filled with joy. I had so much respect and reverence for Dr. Fu as a healer and professor because of her expertise in acupuncture and Chinese herbs, as well as her passion for helping others. She had been my favorite teacher at Five Branches University, and now it had all come full circle because Dr. Fu had learned something from me.

Later, I couldn't help but wonder, *what if I hadn't listened to my inner guidance?* If I had asked someone else to review the book, this amazing and beautiful experience would never have happened. The student would never have been given the opportunity to give back to the teacher.

You see, this is how the Universe works. We are all interconnected. When you practice listening to your inner voice, it will connect you with others who are also listening to their inner voices. This will lead you to opportunities and experiences that your mind could never imagine.

This interconnectedness is like a grove of banyan trees. These trees begin life as a seed growing in the crevices and grooves of *another* tree. A seed lands on a trunk and its emerging roots grow downward into the ground. From the first tree, new seeds are released and spread to nearby trees, and more banyan trees grow.

Eventually, a canopy of trees is formed. The branches and roots in the grove overlap and interlace until you can no longer tell one tree from another. Everything is intertwined like a bird's nest.

When you first try listening to your Dragon Spirit, your connection with the Universe may feel like a small seed. But when you practice quieting your mind regularly, you grow branches and roots just like a banyan tree. Practice until it becomes second *nature*.

Bonus Strategy: Don't Play to Win. Play for Fun.

Okay, this is a bonus strategy because it doesn't really fit in with martial arts. But it's what we tell our kids when they're playing sports—and it's the easiest and most powerful strategy of all. Forget about winning at life or striving to be successful. Simply play for fun.

When you play, you reconnect with your inner child who is free, happy, exuberant, and adventurous. Dance as if no one is watching. Color with crayons. Play with imaginary friends. Make up stories. This playful energy is at the heart of your Dragon Spirit, and it instantly connects you with the energy of the Universe.

In hindsight, I realize this was why I was guided to call my inner wisdom "Dragon Spirit," and why I'm supposed to share it with you this way. You see, the mind's approach to mindfulness is *so serious*. Have you ever been to a meditation class or some other New Age spiritual activity and felt constrained, like you had to be on your best spiritual behavior? No joking, no loud voices, and no disrupting the "om" of the class allowed.

Your inner child, your heart and soul, your Dragon Spirit frankly doesn't give a sh*t about these constraints (by the way, that's the word that rhymes with *sit*, and what I sometimes say when my cat drops a dingleberry in the middle of the living room). When you refer to your inner guidance and soul connection as *Dragon Spirit*, it reminds you that it's not about being serious. Dragon Spirit calls you to adventure, exploration, and play.

Dragon Spirit was certainly calling me when I received an e-mail about the Hay House Writer's Workshop—a weekend event hosted by Hay House, the publishers of this book. In their Writer's Workshops, Hay House teaches aspiring authors how to get their books published and out into the world. I remember being so excited when I learned about the workshop contest where attendees could submit a book proposal, and the grand prize was a publishing contract with Hay House!

However, when I was putting together my book proposal, I struggled for months. Being a Hay House author had been on my bucket list for years, so achieving this goal represented a monumental expansion for me. It was too big a change for my mind to readily accept, so I created a lot of resistance.

Somehow I forgot to sign up for the workshop. I thought I had registered when I hadn't actually done so. Luckily, the Universe intervened and reminded me through a Facebook connection to sign up.

We were given half a year to complete our book proposals, but I procrastinated for months. My mind worried that I wasn't good enough to be a Hay House author, or that I didn't have it in me to write a good book. I didn't know what I would write about. I was intimidated by how accomplished some of my fellow contestants were. How could I compete against them?

I recognized that my mind was out of control with being in control. I was trying to create a book proposal as if it were an essay that I had to hand in for a school assignment—not very fun at all.

Because I recognized this about my mind, I focused instead on releasing any attachment to the outcome. I simply surrendered. I knew that if I couldn't write from a place of alignment and flow, I wasn't writing from my heart. And if I wasn't writing the words from my soul, there was no point in writing the book at all.

I made peace with the idea that I would *not* submit a book proposal. I was okay if my dreams of becoming a Hay House author didn't materialize with this opportunity. What mattered more was how I felt in the moment. Writing had to feel good, and if it didn't, then I was better off doing nothing.

So I gave myself permission to do nothing. As a second generation Chinese Canadian, this was a huge accomplishment for me to be okay with not accomplishing anything at all. It's simply not done. You have to be busy. You have to work hard, or you have to have a really good excuse not to, such as a car accident or being pregnant.

All my life, I had felt compelled to be productive, but suddenly I no longer had to. Instead, I focused on playing. I built toy brick creations with my son. I tried tufting with felt wool and made a lopsided purple dolphin. I doodled with crayons and markers. I read trashy, paranormal teenage romance novels and binged on reality TV cooking shows. I made up stories. I sang and danced.

And then a surprising thing happened. My mind was so preoccupied with doing nothing that I experienced more moments of stillness. And in those moments in between a busy life as a full-time mom running a part-time business, I started to receive downloads from the Universe for my book proposal. A potential book title came to me while showering. As I chopped onions for dinner, I figured out how to structure my chapters.

And when I sat down to write my book proposal, I completed the entire document in four days. There was no way I could have done that if I hadn't been plugged into the wisdom of the Universe. The words flowed through me because I had quieted my mind through play.

So while I'm giving you a Dragon Spirit playbook of strategies, I hope you take away the most important strategy, which is right in the word *play*book. I promise if you play more, you'll feel happier and more joyful, your creativity levels will soar, and you will be able to hear your heart and soul more clearly. And as you do, you will love yourself more and love your life more. And from this, health and vitality will flow.

CHAPTER 17

FINDING AND FOLLOWING YOUR SOUL'S CALLING

Following your heart and soul is the most important catalyst, not only for healing your body, but for leading a life you love. In this chapter, I will share the final leg of my healing journey and reveal how the third and most powerful catalyst changed my life—and how it can transform yours, too.

As you listen to your inner guidance more frequently, you will witness improvements in your health and vitality. You will notice yourself feeling happier and more joyful, but there is one caveat.

You'll also feel a sense of restlessness, as if you need to make a few changes in your life. Perhaps you're feeling this way already. If you are, there's no need to be alarmed. What you are feeling is your Dragon Spirit guiding you to follow your soul's calling. It's your time now—not tomorrow or next week.

You see, if you ignore the restlessness and stay put exactly as you are, you'll be blocking your qi again, and this can cause health issues to reappear. Believe me when I tell you that I speak from personal experience. My life was like a bad movie franchise— *Listen to Your Heart and Then Ignore It, Parts I, II,* and *III.*

Fortunately, you don't need to experience three health crises like I did. You can start following your passion today—right now. Get ready to unleash your sense of adventure and exploration so that you can create your soul's calling. When you do, you clear the energetic blocks in your body, and your life flows abundantly and expansively. You set yourself free to soar.

This chapter is about following your passion and dreaming bigger. It's about addressing fears so that you're not afraid of failing. The only "failing" that exists is the failure to dream big enough. You are on your way now, and it's time for you to become the amazing and brilliant creator that your soul knows you to be. If I can do it, you can, too!

My Story: How I Found My Soul's Calling

As a teenager, I watched my friends and classmates home in on their career choices while I remained uncommitted. I didn't feel I had the option to do what I loved for a living, but even without that constraint, I knew there was something different about me.

I loved art, business, fashion, and writing. I also cared deeply about the environment. But when I saw friends who were *really passionate* about what they were doing, I couldn't muster the same degree of enthusiasm. Sure, I enjoyed an activity, but I never felt like I could devote my entire living, breathing, waking identity to it.

When I compared myself with others, I wondered if I was missing a sense of depth. How could I claim to "love" a subject if I didn't feel as committed to it as others? No matter how much I enjoyed something, I always felt like I could walk away from it if something more interesting caught my attention.

While in university, I dated someone who was studying to become an architect. I admired his singular focus on his chosen vocation and wondered why I couldn't seem to find the one thing that I was passionate about. Interestingly, this feeling followed me through eight full-time jobs, over a half dozen business ventures, and even while I was enrolled in a master's program for Traditional Chinese Medicine.

Before TCM school, I blamed this feeling on not pursuing my interests. However, while I was enrolled in the master's program, I couldn't use the old excuse any longer. I simply couldn't explain why I never got obsessed about things in the same way others could. I could never shake the question, is this all there is to life?

It all came to a head one day while I was at a friend's Christmas party. I was holding my then four-month-old son in my arms while having a conversation with a woman whom I had just met. When she asked me what I did, I told her that I was enrolled in acupuncture school. She was thrilled and gushed, "You must be so passionate about it!"

Her entire face lit up as she awaited my reply. As I took in her unbridled enthusiasm and expectant expression, I realized I wasn't that passionate about it. What could I say to her? Meh? Instead, I plastered on a fake smile, nodded my head, and replied, "Uh, yeah I am." But I wasn't.

A few weeks later, I withdrew from the master's program, even though I had already successfully completed two years of the four-year degree. I knew it was the right choice because after I submitted the paperwork, I floated down the hallway in bliss.

In hindsight, I now realize that I enrolled in the program because I wanted to understand the fundamentals of Chinese Medicine to better understand Chinese reflexology. I wasn't interested in sticking needles in people or prescribing herbs. At the time, though, I wondered if TCM wasn't what I was meant to do, what was my calling?

The answer came to me in an unexpected and unpredictable way.

For the next couple of years after withdrawing from the program, I focused on raising my baby boy. When he was a little over two years old, I signed up for a weekend seminar that was supposed to help me find my calling. Ironically, I didn't find my calling there, but I did discover something even more amazing and transformational.

During the seminar, there was an exercise where we had to work with a partner. We were asked to come up with a list of questions to help us gain insights into the people we were being called to serve. While one partner asked questions, the other was supposed to answer by "channeling" the other person's "target audience." We were advised not to get too hung up over the word *channeling*, but to answer as best as we could.

When it was my turn to answer questions, a sense of hyper-awareness came over me. The room appeared brighter, and I could hear everything with incredible clarity. As I responded to my partner's questions, I felt like the answers were coming from outside of myself—to the left of me, to be precise. It freaked me out.

But the answers I gave were spot on in their accuracy. Later that evening, I decided to try this channeling thing for myself at home. There was one question from the seminar that I was unable to answer so I thought, why not try channeling the answer?

I waited until my husband had gone to sleep because I didn't want him to see me do this weird thing of talking to myself. I sat in the dark and asked my question out loud: "What is the name of my program?"

Even though I was hopeful, I didn't really expect an answer. But right after I asked my question, I started to speak in a strange ethereal voice. The answer I received was "Release Your Dragon Spirit."

I felt so much power and resonance with these words. I realized that everyone has a voice within that is craving to be expressed. But we hold back our voices. We tamp down on our passions. We discount the "little" voice within—shushing it and ignoring it when what we really want to do is roar. Releasing your Dragon Spirit is about sharing your voice with the world to express your brilliance.

As I continued to speak out loud, I surprised myself by giving specific details on how to proceed—everything from dates and numbers to who to contact and what to do. When I acted on the information that I received, I didn't experience my usual struggle of trying to figure out the best plan of action. In fact, I only encountered roadblocks when I was overthinking things.

However, when I followed my gut feeling, everything flowed easily, effortlessly, and expansively.

My mind couldn't help but notice that listening to my inner guidance was actually more effective and more productive. As a result, I made a conscious decision to follow my heart, and from that day onward, my life and health completely transformed. Releasing my Dragon Spirit led me to discover the third catalyst for health and vitality, which is to follow your heart and soul.

I used to think I was reasonably healthy, but when I opened the doors to following my heart, I discovered a new level of vitality. It was like being asleep and then waking up with a new consciousness—or living in the flat plane of a two-dimensional world, only to discover that reality exists in three dimensions, or possibly four or five.

As I saw my life more clearly, both emotionally and spiritually, my eyes healed themselves completely from the early stage macular degeneration. I was guided to follow exercises and activities that helped my eyes grow stronger. I shifted how I thought about myself. I stopped burying things I didn't want to see under the carpet and instead faced them so that I could make positive changes in my life. I also finally acknowledged my brilliance.

When I went to see a new optometrist and mentioned the macular degeneration diagnosis, he meticulously examined my eyes and pronounced that they were perfectly healthy. Not only did the previous "incurable" condition reverse itself, but my eyesight improved, too. The optometrist reduced my eyeglass prescription by about 15 percent. Since then, my eyesight has continued to get better. While my friends are getting glasses in their 30s and 40s because they can no longer see things clearly, my vision gets sharper and crisper with each passing year.

Having worn glasses for over three decades, it feels like a miracle to be able to see more clearly—especially to see my son's face in focus from across the kitchen table. I used to be extremely nearsighted, but I've now cut my eyeglass prescription by over 50 percent, and I see myself on the way to restoring 20/20 vision. The clarity that I have gained from following my heart and living my passion inspires me to help others find and follow their passion, too.

What's _Your_ Passion?

I have yet to meet a single person who didn't already know what their passion was. The truth is that you probably _already know_ what you want to do. The problem is that you don't give yourself permission to do it.

So today, you're going to give yourself permission, or at least take steps toward giving yourself permission. But let's first get your mind on board by addressing two of the most common blocks to following your passion:

- Not knowing what your passion is
- Not knowing how to make it happen

How to Find Your Passion

If you don't know what your passion is, there are a couple of reasons why. The first is that you've probably been trying to figure it out with your brain, but that doesn't work so well because you have to _feel_ your way there. Good thing you've been learning how to get in touch with your heart!

However, there's an even bigger reason why you haven't found the one passion that is the be-all and end-all of your existence. It's because there isn't _one_.

Evolution has always created diversity to ensure the survival of a species. When it comes to following your passion, there are two types of people. The first are those who have one passion and believe in a single cause above all others. This group of _specialists_ pursues their passion with a singular focus because they know, with utmost certainty, that this is their calling in life.

If you are a specialist, then you're already living your passion. But if you're still searching for it, then you may belong to the second group of people—the *generalists*. These people find it challenging to devote themselves to one passion because they have so many diverse interests. They're good at many things, but masters of none. And often, they choose to do what they're good at as opposed to what they're passionate about, simply because *one* passion doesn't seem to emerge above the others.

Generalists may also find that their interests are short-lived. They'll start something new, get all excited about it, immerse themselves in it, and then when they reach a certain level of competency, they lose interest and start something new. Generalists are also easily distracted. It's not that they have a short attention span, but that they're very inquisitive and have a keen awareness of everything going on around them. When something intriguing comes along, they can't help but investigate.

Unfortunately, if you're a generalist, society is set up to make you feel like a failure for following your natural disposition. People are defined by their work, and sticking it out has traditionally been rewarded. It's frowned upon to switch jobs frequently or quit school halfway through an expensive degree—especially when the only reason you want to leave is because you're bored. So you struggle and strive your entire life to find the one thing that will allow you to be as committed as everyone else seems to be. And therein lies the problem.

Rather than viewing yourself as fickle and seeing your lack of focus as a weakness, appreciate it as your *strength*. You have a big picture view. You can see the forest *and* the trees. You're good at a lot of different things and can see multiple perspectives and solutions. You're a Renaissance person.

Your life calling does not exist because *you* are the one who is going to create it. Only you have this unique combination of interests, skills, and experience. There is no template or path for you to follow because no one else has created it before. It's up to you to invent it.

I never know how to answer when someone asks me what I do for a living. Am I a healer, teacher, author, reflexologist, *and* Dragon Spirit guide? Or am I a web programmer, graphic designer, market researcher, online entrepreneur, copywriter, woodworker, or video editor? I'm all of these things and I *love* that I am. If I had to do one thing for the rest of my life, I would wither and die, but that I get to do them all is what excites my heart and soul.

If you can relate to being a generalist, appreciate your nature and give yourself permission to follow your *passions*. Even if your current job is as exciting as watching paint dry, know that every one of your interests, skills, and work experiences can be drawn upon to create your own path for following your soul's calling. That's what excites your heart and scares the crap out of your mind!

Knowing How to Make It Happen

Because your path is unique, no one has done it before—no blueprint exists. The good news is that you create your path as you go along, often without even realizing it. Look at what others have done before you, but then pick and choose what *you* like. All you need is a general direction, and as you keep moving toward it, your path will reveal itself to you one step at a time.

Looking back on my life, there was no way that I could ever have known in advance what my path would be for becoming a Hay House author. But everything I did and experienced—even the most boring jobs that seemed completely unrelated—all contributed to me winning their Writer's Workshop contest and securing a book deal.

My business degree and market research experience made it easy for me to pull together the marketing section of my book proposal entry. Writing articles for a cat blog helped me hone my craft as a writer. My years in the Internet industry enabled me to grow an online presence. All of my health crises from *not* following my passion are what made me the perfect person to write a book on health and following your passion.

There was no way I could have known all of this ahead of time. I couldn't have drawn up a plan before proceeding. In fact, I almost quit a month before everything started really taking off. Because I wanted to provide the best for my son, I seriously considered going back to working in high tech, version 4.0. I'm so glad I stayed true to my heart.

The culmination of your life's purpose is right there for you, too. Whatever you're doing right now and whatever you've done in the past, they are all a part of your path. Even though you may just be looking at a tree right now, your forest will come into view.

The only thing you have to do is *give yourself permission* to fly. Move in the general direction of what you are most passionate about. For me, it was health and vitality. Even though I was interested in a lot of different things, when I moved in that direction, everything seemed to fall into place.

You also don't have to quit your day job to follow your passion. Thinking it has to be all or nothing actually holds you back. As a generalist, this is the worst thing you can do because it goes against your nature to commit to just one pursuit.

I wrote my first book about eco-friendly cat toys while I was working over 50 hours a week in a full-time job. I kept a small sketchbook by my bed and composed cat toy "recipes" a few minutes at a time over the course of several months.

Was the book a career changer? No, but it was the first pet project (bad pun intended) that I actually completed. It also led me to creating a cat blog, which became the training ground for my Chinese reflexology website. Where I am today happened one cat toy recipe and one blog article at a time.

Your Soul's Calling

There is one more thing about your life's passion that I'd like to share with you. I received this message from my Dragon Spirit while I was teaching my Chinese reflexology program. It was a message for the students in the course, but it's also a message for everyone reading this book. If you have ever wondered, "What is my life purpose?" here's your answer:

Your soul's calling is to raise consciousness and uplift others.

The beauty in this statement is that anything can be a conduit for raising consciousness and uplifting others. It doesn't matter what you choose. As a generalist, you can do anything. And as you uplift others, you uplift yourself.

You could be a dancer and touch people's souls through the beauty of your dance. You could be a mother influencing the next generation of children. You could be a guy running a convenience store in a small town and uplift your community through your daily interactions with residents (a true story—just look up Avi Gandhi in Levittown).

So pick something. Take what you enjoy doing and use it as your vehicle for raising consciousness. Listen to your heart. If something feels good and you enjoy doing it, then by all means, do it. Focus on the things you love because that's how you grow into doing even bigger things that you love, and that make a difference in the world.

You have the freedom to choose whatever your heart desires because everything you do is a part of your soul's journey.

The Head to Heart Exercise

Of course, your mind is going to want to have a say in your choices. As a generalist, your biggest challenge is that it's hard to choose just one thing, so you end up picking two, three, four, or a dozen things to do. Or, because the choice is so difficult to make, you don't choose anything at all. Your mind is afraid of missing out or making the wrong choice. For me, the idea of doing just one thing feels like a life sentence.

However, speaking from personal experience, if you want to grow something bigger than yourself, it helps to focus on one thing at a time because this enables you to create momentum that will carry you forward. Otherwise, you simply dilute your efforts and your energy. But it's hard to pick just one, so what's the solution?

Enter the Head to Heart exercise. This is one of my favorite techniques for cutting through the mind's clutter to hear what your heart is calling you to do. You can use this exercise to gain clarity for big life decisions, as well as for small day-to-day choices. I use this technique all the time and even used it to write this book.

When you can't figure out where to begin or what to do, the Head to Heart exercise helps you get an answer in less than five minutes. The reason why this exercise works so well is because it helps you set aside your mind and tune in to what your heart wants.

In order to do the Head to Heart exercise, you'll need a couple of sheets of paper (8.5" x 11" or larger) and a pen or pencil. While you can use a digital drawing tool, I find it's better to be hands-on the old school way.

Step 1

On the first sheet of paper, draw a big circle (or oval if you want to get technical) that covers the entire sheet of paper. Then draw a big heart in the middle of the circle. The heart should be about one-quarter to one-third the size of the circle.

Step 2

Figure out what your question is. The words don't matter as much as the intent behind your question. For example, to get started with following your soul's calling, you can ask yourself, "What do I love to do?"

Then brainstorm a list of at least 20 items to answer your question. Write them down on the second sheet of paper. The reason why you need to come up with so many items is because it gives you permission to be wild and crazy and list anything and everything that comes to mind.

If you're having trouble coming up with items, don't judge your answers or evaluate them for feasibility. Remember, you're making a hypothetical list, so the sky really is the limit.

Step 3

After your brainstorm session, go back and number the items on your list. While you can number items in the order that they are listed, sometimes I go in reverse order and even jump around the page just for fun. When you're finished, take note of how many items there are in total.

Step 4

Now take your first sheet of paper with the heart and circle on it. Write the numbers, from one to your list total, anywhere on the page—the numbers can be in the heart, outside of the heart, in the circle, or outside of the circle. Place the numbers wherever you feel like putting them, but do it randomly, quickly, and without thinking too much. Do not refer to your brainstorm list as you write down the numbers.

Interpreting Your Results

Go through your brainstorm list and match up the numbers on your diagram to the items on your list. Start with number one, and as you go through the numbers, take note of where the number was written on the diagram, because this is where the big reveal happens.

Here's what it all means:

- Anything inside the heart is what your heart wants.

- Anything outside of the heart is what your brain is thinking—not your heart.

- If an item isn't in the circle, then your heart really doesn't want to pursue it.

- If there are several items inside the heart, the item that is closest to the center is what your heart wants you to follow right now.

It is important that you honor your heart's choice. Don't change your mind later. Indecisiveness is a sign of resistance from your mind because it is afraid of making a wrong choice. This fear is an illusion. There is no right or wrong. As long as you keep taking small steps forward, you are following your heart's path. And for that, you deserve a big gold star.

CHAPTER 18

Your Joyful Journey

As we near the end of this book, I want to thank you for your trust in choosing me as your guide. But before it is time for me to step away, I have two final gifts to share with you. Both of these exercises can help you connect even more powerfully with the wisdom of your Dragon Spirit so that you can reach new levels of awareness, consciousness, connection, and vitality in your life. These exercises are my parting gifts to help you access the support of the Universe, along with its healing and revitalizing qi.

So go fetch your favorite journal, or at least a few sheets of paper, and a pen.

The First Gift: Interview with the Universe

This gift was given to me a few years ago, and it has enabled me to receive amazing guidance and clarity from the Universe. That's why I want to pay it forward and share it with you.

I received this gift while attending the workshop where I discovered that I could channel the Universe. One of the workshop leaders, Jeffrey Van Dyk, received a download from the Universe just for me.

During the morning session, I was sitting in the audience, and we were asked if we had any big breakthroughs that we wanted to share. Having just discovered that I could channel the Universe, I figured that was noteworthy enough to put up my hand. A mic was quickly ushered to me, and I stood up to address the group.

I shared my story of channeling and when I mentioned the phrase *release your Dragon Spirit,* it was like an electric bolt went through the crowd. Jeffrey was onstage, and right after I said the phrase, his head jerked suddenly. This movement indicated that he was receiving a download from the Universe.

He shared with me the following exercise. It may have morphed a little from its original form as it has evolved along with me. In addition, you may have encountered variations on this exercise from other teachers. Jeffrey told me later that it's a form of journaling based on Carl Jung's work called *active imagination.* However, I wanted to give credit to Jeffrey because he was the one who first taught it to me.

The activity is a bit like autonomic writing in that you hold a pen in your hand and allow the words of the Universe to flow through you. However, where it differs is that your hand is not moving of its own free accord or because of anyone or anything else. This isn't like a Ouija board where you ask a spirit or entity to speak through you.

Instead, it is an exercise to get in touch with your own higher guidance. It helps you allow the words hidden below the surface of your conscious mind to come through.

Sometimes you need an exercise to distance these pearls of wisdom from yourself because it is hard to accept your own brilliance, but you truly *are* brilliant. As you write, trust that the words will come from your higher guidance. Just set aside your mind and let the wisdom flow through you.

Step 1

In your journal or on a sheet of paper, write your first name followed by a colon at the top of the page. Then compose your message to the Universe. Maybe you have a question, or perhaps there is something that you need to get off your chest. The Universe is a good listener and gives awesome advice.

Step 2

After writing your comment or question, the next step is for the Universe to answer you. On the next line, write *Universe,* or your chosen name for your higher guidance, followed by a colon. If you believe in angels or guides, you can also write down the name of your chosen angel or guide.

I use *DS,* which is short for Dragon Spirit. Sometimes, though, when I want to channel wisdom specific to my business, I write down the name *Ainsley.* I use this name when I want to channel my inner business consultant for practical advice, like where to host my website or what my online workshop schedule will be for the next six months.

Step 3

Start writing. All you have to do is write down the words as you "think" them. Allow your stream of consciousness to flow, and write whatever comes to mind. Don't censor your words even if they don't make much sense. The point is to keep writing without judgment so that you give yourself the freedom to dig deeper and release the answers within.

You don't have to analyze whether the words are from you or the Universe. It doesn't matter, as essentially, the words are all coming from your higher consciousness, which is the same thing as the Universe. Just keep writing. You can even pretend that you're channeling if that helps you set aside your mind and allow the words to flow more freely. There's no right or wrong, just write. Ha!

Step 4

Repeat steps 1 to 3 until you have your own dialogue going on with the Universe. It should look like a magazine interview. Here's an example of what I wrote for myself.

Holly: What can I do right now to make my book a *New York Times* bestseller?

DS: Let go of attachment to the achievement. It doesn't matter how many copies you sell. What matters more is how deeply you touch people's lives. When you reach into someone's soul and help them reconnect to their own brilliance, then you have created something more brilliant and expansive than a fleeting mention on a bestseller list.

Damn, that's good advice!

The Second Gift: Joy Journaling

The second gift I would like to share with you is joy journaling—my take on a gratitude journal. The first time I tried making a list of all the things that I was grateful for, my mind approached the activity like a to-do list. My brain was so used to being efficient and productive that I found myself rushing to come up with a list of ten items. As a result, I suspected that I wasn't receiving the full benefit of practicing gratitude.

Fortunately, I found a way to make it work for me by adding a few small tweaks to the process. I'd love to share these with you because joy journaling has profoundly changed my life. This activity has raised my levels of happiness, consciousness, and creativity to new heights. I also believe it contributed greatly to my winning of the Hay House Writer's Workshop.

As someone with a strong mind, I realized there was one ingredient missing in my previous attempts at practicing gratitude—*feeling*. Joy journaling helps us thinker types tune in to the powerful energy of our hearts. Practicing this activity daily can help you get in touch with your feelings so that you can welcome more love from the Universe.

How to Joy Journal

As soon as you wake up, write in your joy journal. It only takes 5 to 10 minutes and it's worth the time investment because it sets the tone for your entire day. I find that the effects are cumulative—the longer you do this practice, the more benefit you receive.

So, you're going to make a list of ten things that you love and appreciate. This is similar to the standard practice of daily gratitude, but there's a twist. For each item, do the following:

- Write it as a sentence that begins with, *I love and appreciate* . . .

- After listing what you love and appreciate, the next thing you'll write is *Feeling* . . .

- Then tune in to your heart and body to identify what you feel when you think about what you love and appreciate.

- Write that feeling down.

Here are a few examples:

- I love and appreciate my son. Feeling much love and so blessed.

- I love and appreciate that I rode ten miles on my bike. Feeling strong and healthy.

- I love and appreciate my new loft/office space. Feeling clear, calm, and expansive.

By identifying your emotions, you get to reexperience them. This changes the activity from a mental exercise into one that puts you in touch with your feelings. Since emotions are often ignored when you're in thinking mode, this is a powerful way to help you acknowledge (and love and appreciate) your feelings. You're activating positive feelings and vibrations so that you can attract more of the same into your life. Plus, this is awesome for your qi!

Parting Words

Okay, now we really are at the end of the book. It has been my pleasure, delight, and honor to be a part of your journey. And if you would like to continue this journey together and learn more about Chinese reflexology, I would love and appreciate it—you can learn how in the Resources section. Feeling blessed!

So while this book is coming to a close, it is not the end of your journey—rather it is just the beginning. Like the waxing and waning of yin and yang, you have simply reached the end of one phase and are at the cusp of a new beginning. The road has been paved for the amazing and incredible next leg of your journey. You now have the knowledge and tools to take command of your health and step forward in pursuing your passions.

Always remember to follow your heart, listen to your body, and approach each day with the energy of playfulness. It's time to release *your* Dragon Spirit.

Your joyful journey continues . . .

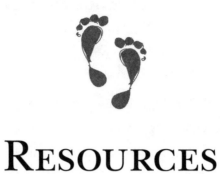

RESOURCES

Chinese Reflexology Foot Charts

On the following pages, you'll find charts that show you where to locate all of the Chinese reflexology points on your feet. There are four charts in total:

1. Chinese Reflexology Points on the Soles

2. Chinese Reflexology Points on the Tops of the Feet

3. Chinese Reflexology Points on the Inside Edges of the Feet

4. Chinese Reflexology Points on the Outside Edges of the Feet

I've included the charts in this book to satisfy your curiosity, but I would caution against massaging points that you haven't yet learned—especially those for the digestive and excretory systems, as it is very important to practice them correctly.

Rather than load up on knowledge, it's better to get into the habit of practicing what you've already learned. When you practice the two routines from Chapter 15 regularly and consistently, they can help your body heal in a balanced and holistic fashion.

A Special Note About Hand Charts

A number of readers who are unable to reach their feet due to injury or other mobility issues have asked me if I have hand charts for the Chinese reflexology points. Unfortunately, I don't have these, but as you learned with the Large Intestine point on your left hand, the reflexology points on the feet map very similarly to those on your hands. In addition, many parts of your body are a microcosm for the body as a whole. There's even a branch of acupuncture called *auricular acupuncture* where healing points for the entire body are located on your ears.

If you find it hard to reach your feet due to a lack of flexibility, I would recommend gentle stretching every day to increase your range of motion. In the meantime, enlist a friend or family member to help you out. You can trade foot massages. It's a fun way to heel—bad pun intended!

1. Chinese Reflexology Points on the Soles

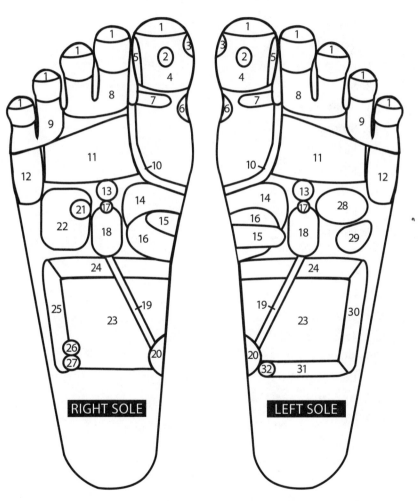

Chinese Reflexology Points on the Soles

1. Sinus
2. Pituitary Gland
3. Nose
4. Brain
5. Temporal Area
6. Parathyroid
7. Neck
8. Eye
9. Ear
10. Thyroid
11. Lung
12. Shoulder
13. Solar Plexus
14. Stomach
15. Pancreas
16. Duodenum
17. Adrenal Gland
18. Kidney
19. Ureter Tube
20. Bladder
21. Gall Bladder
22. Liver
23. Small Intestine
24. Transverse Colon
25. Ascending Colon
26. Ileocecal Valve
27. Appendix
28. Heart
29. Spleen
30. Descending Colon
31. Sigmoid Colon
32. Rectum/Anus

2. Chinese Reflexology Points on the Tops of the Feet

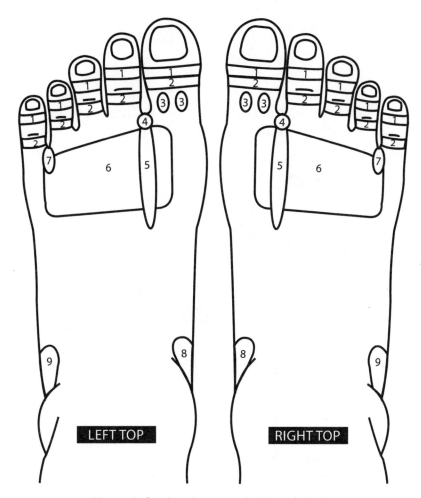

Chinese Reflexology Points on the Tops of the Feet

1. Upper Jaw/Teeth
2. Lower Jaw/Teeth
3. Tonsil/Throat
4. Throat
5. Lymphatic Drainage
6. Breast

7. Inner Ear/Semicircular Canals
8. Lower Lymph Nodes
9. Upper Lymph Nodes

3. Chinese Reflexology Points on the Inside Edges of the Feet

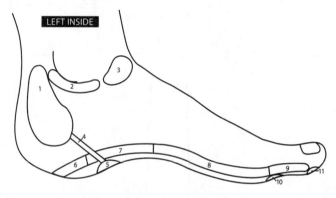

Chinese Reflexology Points on the Inside
Edges of the Feet (left and right feet are the same)

1. Uterus/Prostate
2. Inner Hip
3. Lower Lymph Nodes
4. Ureter Tube
5. Bladder
6. Coccyx and Sacrum
7. Lumbar Spine
8. Thoracic Spine
9. Cervical Spine
10. Parathyroid
11. Nose

4. Chinese Reflexology Points
on the Outside Edges of the Feet

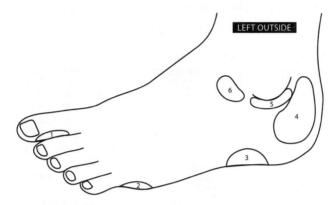

Chinese Reflexology Points on the Outside
Edges of the Feet (left and right feet are the same)

1. Temporal Area

2. Shoulder

3. Knee

4. Ovary/Testicle

5. Outer Hip

6. Upper Lymph Nodes

QUICK REFERENCE TABLE FOR CORE ROUTINE #1

Please refer to the relevant chapters for full details on how to locate and massage these points. Please also review Chapter 7 for important guidelines and precautions.

Chinese Reflexology Core Routine 1*

POINT	LOCATION	TECHNIQUE
1. Kidney Ch. 8	• On soles of both feet, primarily in upper inside quadrant • Below ball of foot and above horizontal halfway line • Thumb width oval with 2/3 in inside quadrant and 1/3 in outside	Massage up and down with thumb, or press and hold with knuckle for 2 to 3 seconds as you move across the point. Apply lubricant if using knuckle. **30 to 60 seconds per foot**
2. Bladder Ch. 8	• Thumb width circle on both feet • Half on inside edge and half on sole • At intersection of where skin meets sole and top edge of heel	Massage up and down with thumb or knuckle. Apply lubricant if using knuckle. **30 seconds per foot**
3. Brain Ch. 9	• On big toe pad of both feet	Massage up and down with thumb. **30 seconds per foot**
4. Temporal Area Ch. 9	• On inside edge of big toe for both feet	Apply lubricant and massage side to side with thumb from tip of toe to base of toe. Reposition thumb at toe tip and repeat. **30 seconds per foot**
5. Lung Ch. 12	• On soles of both feet • Area on ball of foot below three middle toes	Use thumbs to press and massage in small circles, working your way across and down point. **30 to 60 seconds per foot**

POINT	LOCATION	TECHNIQUE
6. Shoulder Ch. 13	• On soles of both feet • Rectangular area under pinky toe, extends to outside edge of foot	Massage up and down with thumb. **15 to 30 seconds per foot**
7. Solar Plexus Ch. 10	• On soles of both feet • Small circle on or near vertical center line, below ball of foot	Massage in small circles or press and twist with knuckle. **15 seconds per foot**
8. Stomach Ch. 10	• On soles of both feet • Circular area below ball of foot on inside edge • Beside Kidney point	Massage top portion up and down with thumb. **15 seconds per foot**
9. Heart Ch. 9	• On sole of left foot • Oval-shaped area in top right quadrant below ball of foot • Beside Kidney point	Massage up and down with thumb. **20 seconds**
10. Spleen Ch. 10	• On sole of left foot • "Blob" in top right quadrant above horizontal halfway line	Massage up and down with thumb or knuckle. Apply lubricant if using knuckle. **30 to 60 seconds**
11. Throat Ch. 14	• On tops of both feet • Small circle in webbing between first two toes	Press and twist with knuckle. **15 seconds per foot**
12. Lymphatic Drainage Ch. 8	• On tops of both feet in webbing between first and second toes	Apply lubricant and stroke with knuckle in downward direction only. **15 to 20 strokes per foot**

*Please refer to Chapter 7 for important guidelines and precautions, and Chapter 15 for details on how to practice this routine.

QUICK REFERENCE TABLE FOR CORE ROUTINE #2

Please refer to the relevant chapters for full details on how to locate and massage these points. Please also review Chapter 7 for important guidelines and precautions.

Chinese Reflexology Core Routine 2*

POINT	LOCATION	TECHNIQUE
1. Kidney Ch. 8	• On soles of both feet, primarily in upper inside quadrant • Below ball of foot and above horizontal halfway line • Thumb width oval with 2/3 in inside quadrant and 1/3 in outside	Massage up and down with thumb, or press and hold with knuckle for 2 to 3 seconds as you move across the point. Apply lubricant if using knuckle. **30 to 60 seconds per foot**
2. Adrenal Gland Ch. 11	• On soles of both feet • Small circle on top of Kidney point	Press and twist with knuckle. **15 seconds per foot**
3. Bladder Ch. 8	• Thumb width circle on both feet • Half on inside edge and half on sole • At intersection of where skin meets sole and top edge of heel	Massage up and down with thumb or knuckle. Apply lubricant if using knuckle. **30 seconds per foot**
4. Inner Hip Ch. 13	• On inside edge of both feet • "Breakfast sausage" below and behind anklebone	Apply lubricant and massage back and forth with thumb. **15 to 30 seconds per foot**
5. Uterus/ Prostate Ch. 14	• Teardrop-shaped area on inside edge of both feet • Located below and behind anklebone	Apply lubricant and massage up and down with knuckle. **15 seconds per foot**
6. Pituitary Gland Ch. 11	• Small circle In center of big toe pad of both feet • Slightly closer to inside edge of foot	Press and twist with knuckle. **15 seconds per foot**

POINT	LOCATION	TECHNIQUE
7. Liver Ch. 11	• Square on sole of right foot in top left quadrant • Left of Kidney point, below ball of foot and above horizontal halfway line	Massage up and down with thumb or knuckle. Apply lubricant when using knuckle. **15 seconds**
8. Gall Bladder Ch. 12	• On sole of right foot • Small circle in top right quadrant of Liver point	Press and twist with knuckle. **15 seconds**
9. Knee Ch. 13	• On outside edge of both feet • In depression above heel where skin meets sole	Use thumb or knuckle to massage back and forth. Apply lubricant when using knuckle. **15 to 30 seconds per foot**
10. Outer Hip Ch. 13	• On outside edge of both feet • "Breakfast sausage" below and behind anklebone	Apply lubricant and massage back and forth with index finger **15 to 30 seconds per foot**
11. Ovary/ Testicle Ch. 14	• Teardrop shaped area on outside edge of both feet • Located below and behind anklebone	Apply lubricant and massage up and down with knuckle **15 seconds per foot**

*Please refer to Chapter 7 for important guidelines and precautions, and Chapter 15 for details on how to practice this routine.

MINI REFLEXOLOGY ROUTINES

The reflexology points that you've learned in this book can be used in various combinations to give your qi a boost or to help with short-term health concerns. Here are a dozen powerful mini reflexology routines for the following conditions and purposes:

1. Brain boost
2. Common cold remedy and prevention
3. Constipation
4. Detoxing the body
5. Energy boost
6. Headaches and migraines
7. Indigestion
8. Insomnia
9. Knee pain
10. Seasonal allergy symptoms
11. Sore throat
12. Stress, worry, and overthinking

Important Guidelines

Don't try to practice all of the mini routines together. You can, however, choose one mini routine to massage once a day in addition to the core reflexology routines (unless otherwise noted).

If a reflexology point appears in both routines, it's not necessary to massage it twice. Simply check which routine has the longest time specified, and massage the point for that length of time.

Even though mini routines consist of only a handful of points, they're very powerful, so the precautions from Chapter 7 apply, including not practicing on yourself if you are pregnant or if you have an acute heart condition. As long as you follow the routines as instructed, it is highly unlikely that you will trigger detox symptoms in your body.

However, if you do notice anything out of the ordinary, stop massaging your feet, and only resume again when you're feeling back to normal (see Chapter 7 for details on detox symptoms). If your health issue persists, please see your medical practitioner.

1. Brain Boost

This routine helps improve circulation of qi and blood to the brain. Massage the following points daily.

- Brain, 60 seconds
- Temporal area, 30 seconds
- Kidney, 60 seconds

2. Cold Remedy and Prevention

Use this routine on its own to help get over a cold faster and reduce the likelihood of catching one in the first place. Practice this routine four times a day until you are feeling better. Then reduce to twice a day for two additional days. Practice this routine exclusively and resume the core routines when your symptoms have passed.

- Lung, 60 seconds
- Sinus*, 30 seconds
- Throat/tonsil*, 30 seconds
- Throat, 20 to 30 seconds
- Lymphatic drainage, 30 strokes

*You'll find instructions for these points, a detailed description of this routine, and a downloadable quick reference chart at www.chinesefootreflexology.com/coldremedy.

3. Constipation

For temporary constipation due to tension or unsavory bathroom conditions, practice this mini routine. Massage the points and then take a deep breath and relax your abdominal cavity for 15 to 30 seconds. Repeat until a bowel movement occurs, or up to a maximum of five times in one bathroom session. If your constipation persists or is accompanied by blood, see your doctor.

- Large Intestine (on hand), 15 strokes
- Anus/rectum (on hand), 15 seconds

4. Detoxing the Body

For gentle detoxification over time, massage the following points daily.

- Kidney, 60 seconds
- Bladder, 30 seconds
- Lymphatic drainage, 15 strokes

5. Energy Boost

This routine helps to recharge your qi over time. Massage the following points daily.

- Kidney, 60 seconds
- Adrenal, 15 seconds
- Spleen, 30 seconds
- Lung, 30 seconds

6. Headaches and Migraines

Practice this routine for pain relief from headaches and migraines. Massage the following points as needed up to three times a day.

- Temporal area, 60 seconds
- Liver 3*, 60 seconds
- Large Intestine 4*, 60 seconds
- Gall Bladder 41*, 30 to 60 seconds
- Face*, 30 to 60 seconds

* You'll find instructions for these points, a detailed description of this routine, and a downloadable quick reference chart at www.chinesefootreflexology.com/painfree.

7. Indigestion

Ease cramps and bloating from temporary indigestion with this routine. Massage the following points twice a day. Practice this routine exclusively and resume the core routines when symptoms have passed.

- Stomach, 30 seconds
- Spleen, 60 seconds
- Large Intestine (on hand), 30 strokes

8. Insomnia

Fall asleep more easily and sleep better with this routine. Massage the following points at night before sleep. You can also massage them if you wake up in the middle of the night. Daily practice of this routine can also help you sleep better over time.

- Kidney, 60 seconds
- Heart, 20 seconds
- Spleen, 30 seconds
- Liver 2*, 60 seconds
- Heart 7*, 60 seconds

*You'll find instructions for these points and a detailed description of this routine at: www.chinesefootreflexology.com/sleep.

9. Knee Pain

For knee pain due to injury or overuse, massage this point (on the same foot as the painful knee) three times a day until the knee is feeling better.

- Knee, 60 seconds

If you have a history of chronic knee issues, add the following point:

- Kidney (both feet), 60 seconds

10. Seasonal Allergy Symptoms

For relief of seasonal allergy symptoms, massage the following points daily.

- Lung, 60 seconds
- Sinus*, 60 seconds
- Nose, 30 seconds
- Throat, 20 to 30 seconds
- Eyes*, 30 to 60 seconds
- Lymphatic drainage, 30 strokes

*You'll find instructions for these points, a detailed description of this routine, and a downloadable quick reference chart at www.chinesefootreflexology.com/allergies.

11. Sore Throat

This routine helps give you pain relief from a sore throat. Practice this routine exclusively and resume the core routines when symptoms have passed. Massage the following points every hour for four to six hours.

- Throat, 60 seconds
- Throat/tonsil*, 60 seconds

*You'll find instructions for these points, a detailed description of this routine, and a downloadable quick reference chart at www.chinesefootreflexology.com/sorethroat.

12. Stress, Worry, and Overthinking

To help calm the mind and release worry, massage the following points daily.

- Brain, 30 seconds
- Temporal area, 30 seconds
- Spleen, 30 seconds
- Liver 3*, 60 seconds
- Heart 7*, 60 seconds

*You'll find instructions for these points and a detailed description of this routine at www.chinesefootreflexology.com/calm.

MORE WAYS TO LEARN

Amazing Feet *Newsletter and Free Articles*

Visit my website to sign up for a complimentary "monthly" e-mail newsletter. It's a fun way to learn self-healing tips and techniques for the body, mind, heart, and spirit. *Monthly* is in quotes because I aim for monthly, but sometimes send out the newsletter less than once a month.

Since I am a full-time mom, life can get pretty hectic, so it all depends on whether we're visiting family in Canada, if there's a little boy's birthday party in the works, or other family stuff going on. In rare instances, I may send the newsletter out twice a month if I've had a recent streak of productivity and have a lot of information to share.

When you sign up for my newsletter, you'll also receive downloadable Chinese reflexology foot charts and a series of mini online lessons. While much of the information in the lessons is covered in this book, they're a great way to review what you've learned so far—plus there's a video, too.

I'll also send out the occasional message to let you know about upcoming online classes, for which you'll receive exclusive savings. As a busy mom, I promise that you won't get tons of e-mail from me. I also promise to keep your e-mail address confidential and to only send you messages that are full of useful and valuable information.

My website is also a great resource for free articles on Chinese reflexology, TCM, the mind-body connection, and tips and advice on following your passion.

Get your complimentary newsletter and read free articles at www.chinesefootreflexology.com.

Chinese Reflexology Sole Mastery Program

This groundbreaking program is designed to take your healing journey to the next level:

- Learn how to use a reflexology stick.
- Confidently locate and massage all of the points in traditional Chinese reflexology.
- Release your Dragon Spirit for life-changing transformation.
- Plus much more!

The Chinese Reflexology Sole Mastery Program is a six-month online program with the option for in-person instruction. I'd love it if our paths meet up again in the future. To learn more, please visit www.chinesefootreflexology.com/learn.

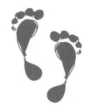

ACKNOWLEDGMENTS

Wow, creating this book has been an incredible journey for me. I would like to thank the following people for their assistance and support in helping me to manifest my brilliance.

Dr. Gilbert Tay, thank you for helping me recover my health, teaching me this amazing system of healing, and being so generous in sharing Chinese reflexology with the world to alleviate suffering. Dr. Ning X. Fu, thank you for being an amazing and inspiring teacher, reviewing my manuscript, providing constructive feedback, and contributing research information.

Leo, thank you for your eagle eyes and encouragement during the book-writing process, and also during the creation of my book proposal. Dr. Amanda Noelle, thank you for your gift of soul sole. And to the Hay House team, thank you for choosing my book proposal and for your awesome support in creating an amazing book.

Zunaid, thank you for believing in me, cheering me on, being a sounding board, and handling all the family stuff when things were down to the wire and I needed to write. K, thanks for your understanding when Mommy had to write instead of play alligators, monkeys, and snakes with you. I owe you a game of cat telemarketer!

Finally, thank you to all of my blog readers. Without you, this book would not exist. Wishing you amazing health and vitality for your brilliant journey in life!

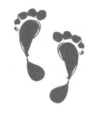

ABOUT THE AUTHOR

Holly Tse is a former high-tech worker turned holistic healer, teacher, author, and Dragon Spirit Guide. In addition to wearing many hats, she is also a full-time mom. Holly is the founder of ChineseFootReflexology.com, the premier English language website on Chinese reflexology, with readers from over 200 countries worldwide.

As a Chinese Canadian, Holly followed cultural expectations by getting good grades in school and a good job when she graduated. She worked in the corporate world until her body spoke up by breaking down. She then walked away from a ten-year career to follow her heart and soul. As a result, she healed her body and discovered the secrets of amazing health and vitality. It is her passion and joy to share them with you!

Holly lives in Northern California with her husband, son, and mischievous cat. She enjoys biking, swimming, tasty food, and the occasional reality TV cooking show.

Hay House Titles of Related Interest

YOU CAN HEAL YOUR LIFE, the movie,
starring Louise Hay & Friends
(available as a 1-DVD program and an expanded 2-DVD set)
Watch the trailer at: www.LouiseHayMovie.com

THE SHIFT, the movie,
starring Dr. Wayne W. Dyer
(available as a 1-DVD program and an expanded 2-DVD set)
Watch the trailer at: www.DyerMovie.com

destressifying: The Real-World Guide to Personal
Empowerment, Lasting Fulfillment, and Peace of Mind, by davidji

Life Loves You: 7 Spiritual Practices to Heal Your Life,
by Louise Hay and Robert Holden, Ph.D.

Living Pain-Free: Natural and Spiritual
Solutions to Eliminate Physical Pain,
by Doreen Virtue and Robert Reeves, N.D.

Medical Medium: Secrets Behind Chronic and Mystery
Illness and How to Finally Heal, by Anthony William

Out of the Blue: True-Life Experiences of Awakening,
Revelation, and Transformation, by Mary Terhune

All of the above are available at your local
bookstore, or may be ordered by visiting:

Hay House USA: www.hayhouse.com®
Hay House Australia: www.hayhouse.com.au
Hay House UK: www.hayhouse.co.uk
Hay House South Africa: www.hayhouse.co.za
Hay House India: www.hayhouse.co.in

We hope you enjoyed this Hay House book. If you'd like to receive our online catalog featuring additional information on Hay House books and products, or if you'd like to find out more about the Hay Foundation, please contact:

Hay House, Inc., P.O. Box 5100, Carlsbad, CA 92018-5100
(760) 431-7695 or (800) 654-5126
(760) 431-6948 (fax) or (800) 650-5115 (fax)
www.hayhouse.com® • www.hayfoundation.org

Published and distributed in Australia by: Hay House Australia Pty. Ltd., 18/36 Ralph St., Alexandria NSW 2015
Phone: 612-9669-4299 • *Fax:* 612-9669-4144 • www.hayhouse.com.au

Published and distributed in the United Kingdom by:
Hay House UK, Ltd., Astley House, 33 Notting Hill Gate, London W11 3JQ
Phone: 44-20-3675-2450 • *Fax:* 44-20-3675-2451 • www.hayhouse.co.uk

Published and distributed in the Republic of South Africa by:
Hay House SA (Pty), Ltd., P.O. Box 990, Witkoppen 2068
info@hayhouse.co.za • www.hayhouse.co.za

Published in India by: Hay House Publishers India,
Muskaan Complex, Plot No. 3, B-2, Vasant Kunj, New Delhi 110 070
Phone: 91-11-4176-1620 • *Fax:* 91-11-4176-1630 • www.hayhouse.co.in

Distributed in Canada by: Raincoast Books,
2440 Viking Way, Richmond, B.C. V6V 1N2 •
Phone: 1-800-663-5714 • *Fax:* 1-800-565-3770 • www.raincoast.com

Take Your Soul on a Vacation

Visit www.HealYourLife.com® to regroup,
recharge, and reconnect with your own magnificence.
Featuring blogs, mind-body-spirit news, and life-changing
wisdom from Louise Hay and friends.

Visit www.HealYourLife.com today

Free e-newsletters
from Hay House, the Ultimate
Resource for Inspiration